Genetics
Isn't Everything

Genetics
Isn't Everything

How to Make Your
'G-E-N-E-S'
Fit You

KATHERINE S. EGAN

outskirts
press

Dedication

I dedicate this book to you, dear reader, and to anyone who has ever felt hopeless, lost, or stuck on a never-ending wheel of medical illness, diagnoses, and treatment. The frustration that comes with not knowing why we feel so sick and tired, and what that means to our future longevity, can drain us of the vibrant lives we were born to live. No matter what you may have been told, know there is another way. Know that you are not destined to have the same health issues as your parents or grandparents. Know that your chronic conditions or incurable illnesses may not be chronic or incurable. Know that you are not alone. Regardless of what you've heard in the past, there may be another, non-medicated way to heal.

I am here to share proof from those who took matters into their own hands. May these individual stories and journeys provide inspiration, and may you find hope in their messages.

Acknowledgements

This book would not exist if not for all the courageous women who bared their souls to me so that I could share their stories with the universe. Whether your story was included or not, you are braver and stronger than you know and I am filled with gratitude for each and every one of you. I hope you find peace in this world and inspiration to keep moving forward.

I am immensely grateful for my husband, Sam. This man knows me better than I know myself. He knows when to leave me to my musings and when to push. Sam does all the food shopping for us and cooks for me every night so that I can focus on writing. He nourishes my body with his cooking, my heart with his love, and my soul with his presence. He always has my back.

I am beyond grateful for Marley and her magical ways. She is truly worth her weight in gold.

Kim, I have no words. Your support, your love, your energy kept me going and continually motivated me to do better.

I am deeply grateful for Sylva, without whom this book would have never started. All the dots link back to her—from "energy, focus, and mental clarity" to nutritional rebalancing to the Institute for Integrative Nutrition (IIN) to this book. She inspires me every day with her light and her passion. Watching her children grow up with the knowledge they have of nutrition is truly wonderful. They will never go down the path of ill health.

I am so appreciative of my mom, who always has loads of love to share through her smile, her warmth, and her baking, even when she's not feeling up to it. Special thanks to Tim, for always being my big brother, to Tina for always trying to keep him healthy, and to George for showing the world you can be happy and grateful even in the worst of circumstances.

For Izzie, Sheryl and Team Heart, I am forever grateful for your never-ending love and support.

Special thanks to Dr. Paul Arciero for writing my foreword. Being an internationally renowned optimal health and performance expert, his research into protein pacing and quality versus quantity of exercise, as well as his understanding about food quality and the importance of eating the right foods at the right time lend much support and credence to my book. I cannot thank him enough for his thoughtful and thought-provoking words.

And last but not least, a special thanks to Trent Herrera and Dana Nelson and the outstanding staff at Outskirts Press who seamlessly helped make my debut book a dream come true.

Foreword

In an era of skyrocketing rates of lifestyle-related diseases we should all be asking ourselves: "To be or not to be healthy?" This question examines our fundamental decision-making process when facing healthy and unhealthy lifestyle choices. For example, do we choose to eat nourishing foods such as fresh vegetables and fruit or do we habitually grab the donut and soda? Or, how about whether to stand up from our chair or couch every hour and take a 5- to 10-minute walk around the house or office building instead of sitting for hours at a time? The first step of a healthy lifestyle begins with daily decisions to choose healthy alternatives over unhealthy ones. In addition, our busy and stressful lives combined with easy access to processed, nutrient-deficient food makes it even more important to choose "healthy."

In writing *Genetics Isn't Everything: How to Make Your "Genes" Fit You*, Katherine Egan poignantly challenges the often-repeated dogma that our inherited genetic makeup is the major factor determining our health and wellness. Challenging this theory, she powerfully illustrates the importance of personal "self-care," nutrition, and daily choices that enhance our genetic code and propel us to optimal wellness versus simply living disease-free.

As a lifelong athlete and an active exercise and nutrition scientist for the past 30-plus years, I've been a devoted "evangelist" for all things fitness, nutrition, health, and wellness in my roles as a consultant, college professor, motivational speaker, business owner, writer, TV and radio personality, and husband and father of three. My research endeavors in nutrition and fitness lifestyle interventions to optimize health and physical performance have resulted in more than 55 peer-reviewed published research papers.

In support of Katherine's work with *Genetics Isn't Everything*, my research consistently demonstrates the effectiveness of high-quality nourishment and exercise training on improving energy metabolism, body composition, glucose tolerance, and cardiovascular disease risk in healthy and diseased populations, particularly among women. As a result of this research, I completely agree with Katherine that we have much more control over our bodies and our health than we may realize. I have specifically focused on markers of cardiovascular risk and cognitive function of adults, but it is fascinating to think about how other biomarkers (such as C-reactive protein, leptin, ghrelin, IGF-1, etc.), thyroid function, endocrine stressors, and all of the hidden illnesses that seem to be multiplying but are not easily diagnosed, can be aided and even healed with the right nutrition and exercise program.

Personally, I can also relate to the frustration of trying to make sense of clinical data versus physical manifestations. After years of experience and research I have developed a one-of-a-kind system called the PRISE protocol (Protein Pacing, Resistance, Interval, Stretching, Endurance) to cut through all the confusing health, performance, and "body transforma-tion" information that's out there. Living each day with a focus on the quality of our meal timing, macronutrient intakes, and exercise training interventions *does* change body composition and numerous health markers ... we *can* take control!

It's difficult to sort through the masses of information, and even leading nutrition scientists are at odds over which diet is the best for us. And there doesn't seem to be an easy winner emerging any time soon. However, there is one common de-nominator among all of these various diets that all nutrition and diet experts agree, and I am the nutrition scientist who developed this nutritional strategy called "Protein Pacing™." For the past decade, I've perfected the technology to maximize the benefits of Protein Pacing™ with my GenioFit™ mobile app. What makes Protein Pacing™ so unique and beneficial is how seamlessly it fits into any diet program. I define Protein Pacing™ as the "right protein at the right time." It's important to me that the years I have spent researching can finally be ap-plied to practical everyday life. The practice of Protein Pacing, and whole food, is key to gaining optimal health.

I, like Katherine, have been fortunate enough to live my entire life without a major illness, and have been fortunate enough to reach peak physical performance goals, but I have seen loved ones and clients suffer, so I think all humans pon-der at some point or another—whether we realize it or not—how much of our health is genetic and how much of it is a result of the daily choices we make.

In the following pages, I'm confident you will find this material inspiring, motivating, and quite frankly illuminating when you read how much Katherine clarifies that genes play a much smaller role in our overall health than the "news" may have us believe. This is an exciting new age. When you read the deeply moving stories of what these women have endured and shared (and she promises a book on children and men next), you begin to realize that you are not alone and that there are many professionals like us who want to serve. Don't give up. Read ahead. I encourage everyone to absorb this information, and if you are short of time, skip forward to the sections that you can relate to the most but, most importantly, reach out to the professionals who are here to help you.

There is always *hope*. Whether it is coaching a pro athlete or an Olympian on nutrition or teaching a yoga class—yes, I'm certified in two styles of yoga—or simply helping others take their personal challenges and past defeats and motivating them to believe they can make change and therefore achieve it, I am a huge proponent of epigenetics and that we can help protect our genes and stay healthy and vibrant to live a longer and healthier life. I also believe in getting outside and appreciating the beauty of nature or taking time to meditate, whether that is running or sitting still.

As a lifelong athlete and dedicated teacher, coach, and scientist, I encourage you to first learn the basics here about genetics and understand that we really have much more control over our destinies than we may be taught. Then, go live the ultimate wellness lifestyle, get outside, explore and achieve peak performance, and take control of your life. As Katherine says, "Genetics isn't everything, so, go and make your 'genes' fit you!"

A new season is upon us all and we deserve the best! This information is invaluable, and the hearts of the people behind this work are sincere. Our lives are made better by helping you. That is what drives us. Life is busy—believe me, I know that—but there is so much value to share and personal stories to back this up that you owe it to yourself to read and to heal.

Best in health and wellness,

Dr. Paul

Dr. Paul J. Arciero, FACSM, FTOS
CEO & President
PRISE LLC and GenioFit
www.geniofit.com
paul@geniofit.com

Dr. Paul J. Arciero, D.P.E., M.Sc., M.Sc., FACSM, FTOS, is a Fellow of the American College of Sports Medicine and The Obesity Society and has served as a member of the Advisory Board for the American Heart Association (Capital Region). He is a leading expert in nutrition and fitness lifestyle interventions to optimize health and physical performance. He has published more than 55 peer-reviewed research studies on performance nutrition and exercise training in the world's most respected science journals, including *Obesity Journal, Frontiers in Physiology, American Journal* of *Preventive Medicine, American Journal of Physiology, Nutrients, Journal of Applied Physiology,* and *American Journal of Clinical Nutrition.* Several of Dr. Paul's publications have attained the coveted "classic" status, being referenced by other scientists at least 100 times in peer-reviewed science/medical journals. One of Dr. Paul's most important scientific discoveries was the observation that consuming ideal amounts of high-quality protein (20–40 grams per serving) 4–6 times per day (with and without exercise training) reduced total body and abdominal fat to a greater extent than three "traditional" higher-carbohydrate meals per day and led to the terms "Protein Pacing" and "PRISE Protocol," as well as numerous additional peer-reviewed publications. Dr. Paul's work is extensively cited in medical publications such as the *American Heart Association (American Heart Association & Dr. Paul), Duke Medicine Health News, Science Daily,* and *Villanova COPE* as well as mainstream popular media, including *The Wall Street Journal, Fox News, Prevention, Good Housekeeping, WebMD, O Magazine, TIME, Huffington Post, Daily Mail, SELF, Glamour, Shape, Health, Women's Health, Women's World, Muscle and Fitness, Men's Fitness,* and *Men's Health.* Other national media outlets include "Doctor Radio XM/Sirius" and "Rusty Lion Podcast" on iTunes. The National Public Radio program *"Academic Minute*: Best of Our Knowledge" has not only featured Dr. Paul's work but also given him the *2015 Most Likely to Change the World Senior Superlative Award.* Dr. Paul has been an invited expert speaker at more than 200 conferences around the world. He regularly serves as a sports performance nutritionist for collegiate (NCAA Div. 1-III), Olympic (cyclists, speed skaters, rowers, biathletes), and professional athletes (National Hockey League – American Hockey League affiliates Adirondack Phantoms, Philadelphia Flyers and Adirondack Flames, Calgary Flames). Dr. Paul is President and CEO of *PRISE LLC*, a nutrition and fitness consulting company that owns the *GenioFit*™ app on iTunes (*GenioFit App*). Dr. Paul is the Director of the Human Nutrition and Metabolism Laboratory and a Full Professor in the Health and Exercise Sciences Department at Skidmore College. In addition, he is an Adjunct Research Professor in the Psychology & Neuroscience Department at Union College and has served as an Adjunct Professor in the Nutrition Department at Sage College. Dr. Paul serves on Scientific Advisory Boards for the nutrition and food industry. Dr. Paul received his undergraduate degree from Central Connecticut State University in 1986, an M.Sc. in exercise physiology from Purdue University in 1987, and an M.Sc. in nutritional sciences from University of Vermont in 1993. He received his doctorate from Springfield College in 1993 with a specialization in nutrition and exercise science and completed post-doctoral fellowship training in applied physiology from Washington University School of Medicine in 1994. He is a former top-ranked collegiate tennis player who also played on the European Satellite tennis circuit. Dr. Paul currently lives in Saratoga Springs, NY, with his beautiful wife Karen and three amazing sons.

Please visit www.geniofit.com, www.proteinpacing.com, #paularciero (Twitter), or Paul J. Arciero (Facebook) for more information on Dr. Paul.

Table of Contents

PART THREE
Invisible Illness: Just Because You Don't See It Doesn't Mean It's Not There

PART FOUR
Illnesses Surfacing On The Skin

PART FIVE
Body Or Mind? When Food Becomes Your Enemy And Not Your Medicine

PART SIX
Changing Your Destiny: Why Genes Don't Have To Have The Final Answer

Introduction

Getting well is easy. It's getting sick that takes years of dedicated hard work.

—Dr. Richard Schulze

They say the only constant is change. Sadly, today, there seems to be another constant: there are many more serious illnesses affecting our population than there were even 60 years ago. It seems as though not one human being, and perhaps not even one pet or animal, makes it through life unscathed. Unfortunately, almost every person and definitely every family (and sometimes multiple members of the same family) seems to suffer from a chronic long-term health issue or terminal illness.

All this suffering takes the thrill out of the optimal life we were supposed to lead. Whether physical or mental disorders, unhealthy relationships, overwork, or too much daily stress, our generation is falling apart at the seams and as a result is damaging the future health of generations to come.

Even in my lifetime, only half a century so far, disease has changed through the years. Whereas there used to be American families that were struck with sudden death by accidents and deaths due to epidemics that came and went, there was never the same widespread malaise that we see today. Why is that? Why are we not holding up as well as we used to? What has changed?

That is exactly what this book explores. I am here to help you see that we are more than our genetic, inherited makeup. We can be more than the sick and tired generation expecting to die of cancer or heart disease. We are more than the toxic and GMO food-poisoned environment we live in. Let me show you what I mean by starting with a little psychological experiment.

Imagine for a moment you are the one the doctor tells has an incurable illness. Incurable. Imagine the fear, the emotions, the helplessness you would immediately feel. Your heart might be palpitating just from the thought. *Incurable* is not a word that anyone ever wants to hear. The word itself rings like the word *cancer*. But other than the fear that the word elicits, the question becomes: do we have any control over an incurable illness and its progression? Is it actually terminal—in other words, a "guaranteed" death sentence—just because the doctor has uttered those precise words? Or instead, is it a chronic condition that at this point doctors just don't seem to know how to cure? Does it even matter? Does this necessarily mean there is no hope?

I propose that it does matter, psychologically. I propose, however, that it is not always the word or diagnosis, but instead it is *how* we think and our willingness to change our current environment that can potentially save our lives and bring us to a new level of health and well-being. This is the hope I bring to you in this book. This is the hope that I share as I spread and disseminate the growing bed of information on epigenetics versus genetics.

Continuing on with the psychological experiment—what would it be like to think of a lifetime diagnosis where you are not terminal but there is no cure? How does that make you feel? Perhaps to some it is a relief that they have longer than three to six months to live. Agreed. However, playing devil's advocate for a moment, have you ever met someone crippled over in pain, unable to move and completely bedridden due to multiple sclerosis (MS) or rheumatic arthritis (RA), or who can't leave the house because of Crohn's disease? Or have you ever heard the term "phantom" illness, where the doctors agree they can't cure you but can only give you a diagnosis code, ICD-9-CM Diagnosis Code 799.9: Other unknown and unspecified cause of morbidity and mortality? Yes, an actual code doctors use for medical billing when they can't figure out what the illness truly is. What does it feel like to think of an entire lifetime with one of the thousands of debilitating diseases that now plague us worldwide? Does this sound like a life to you? Does it make you sad just thinking about it? Does it grieve you looking around at all the sick people in the world and watching your loved ones deal with terminal diseases such as cancer? I know it pains me.

Think about what it is like to live a life connected to pain meds, getting liquid food, perhaps through a feeding tube, and constantly being moved by nurses or a loved one from one spot to another so that sores don't develop, thereby having the opportunity to lie 30 or 40 years this way (because of advanced technologies); is this life? Is this life when you feel so terrible every day, even if you are not confined to your bed, that you can't enjoy one person, your children or mate, or even being in your body because it is wracked with pain or you simply lack the energy to even function. Is this life?

In the end, the type of life I'm talking about in this book is the exact opposite of this pain and tragedy—may I even be so bold as to say some of this unnecessary pain and tragedy? The type of life I am sharing with you is a vibrant and vivacious life, one that you enjoy well before anyone gets to this stage of incurable.

Despite what you are being told by physicians, "Big Pharma," fake news, etc., the diseases we will be looking at in this book rarely move to the confinement stage until many other things have gone awry. Whether the person has been misdiagnosed for years, has been exposed to unknown environmental toxins, ingested toxic food and water, or perhaps missed daily opportunities to summon their immune system, purposefully created to self-protect and heal—our "hidden warriors" per se—we are forced into a diseased life we are told is our only choice. Therefore we live a life going from one pharmaceutical to the next, leading to another set of problems and sometimes serious health consequences, and we feel we have no other options. With this, the downward spiral begins, pulling in friends, family, loved ones all because of the ill person and time involved in care, and as a result, our lives are spent in a worrisome mess versus a blessed gathering ... until death do us part.

You get my point. Why so graphic? Because it is time for all of us to remove the denial, the thinking that oh, that can't happen to me; oh, I can't get pregnant or get AIDS only having had unprotected sex one time; oh, it runs in my family so there is nothing I can do. It is time to start to wake up. Begin to realize that because of the world we live in today, if we don't start setting up and taking our precautions now, get our fighting and hidden protective warriors in line now, help the genes we were born with now, we will simply become another living miserable, unhappy, and doomed statistic.

Think again for a moment about that word *incurable*. Do you ever want to hear that word? Do you ever want to hear the word *cancer*? No, but if that day comes, and even better, before that day comes, what can we do to be proactive? After all, there are cancers that can be removed and a person can recover from, cancers that are treated and go into remission, cancers that can be cured, and, on the other side, unfortunate but true, cancers that swiftly become terminal and take loved ones of all ages away from us far too soon.

Amazingly, there are more people around the world than you realize that have taken their medical news and diagnosis, gone totally against the grain, and have even managed to completely heal themselves. Is it a miracle? Perhaps not. What if instead, our illnesses are progressing due to a lack of proper information? And, what if healing or remission is simpler and quicker than most medical treatments prescribed normally take?

One of the purposes in writing this book is to share the stories of a number of people who transformed their lives to stop from digesting the news that they had an *incurable* illness, a chronic illness, an unknown illness—and the list goes on. They took measures into their own hands. Extraordinarily, a few even found a way to cure their incurable illness, and all found a way to heal into a life that is now enjoyable. This gives us hope. This motivates us to look further, search harder, make changes and find a way to fight through to health.

Our body is designed in such a brilliant way that it is pre-programmed to move toward healing—given the right circumstances. This is what I want to share with you. I want to show you that environment and how we treat our body—in other words epigenetics (which I describe more thoroughly in chapter one)—can influence and boost our system enough that our genes can get support. Instead of moving towards destroying parts of our body, shutting down systems, and deteriorating, our body takes the help we give it and starts to build reinforcements, like a healthy immune system, so that we can get stronger. Our purpose in life is to live happy, fulfilling, and fun lives! We are not supposed to live a passionless, painful, joyless life.

In this book I share stories about people who have changed their health and thus their lives with nutrition, self-care, and self-compassion. A happy and healthy life, while not guaranteed to everyone, is within reach. You can change your health with nutrition. You can take your life back, and I am here to show you how.

Don't get me wrong. I'm not saying we don't need doctors, nurses, surgeons, orthopedists, paramedics, social workers, and all other roles in the medical industry. We do. I have enormous respect for health-care workers. *I have enormous respect for anyone who works to serve others.* I have close family in health-related fields. I know how hard they work and how much they care. I have seen firsthand how compassionate and caring nurses and surgeons and oncologists are. My mother is currently going through radiation and chemotherapy for her fourth distinct cancer. She has had breast cancer twice, stomach cancer where they removed 95% of her stomach, ovarian cancer, and most recently, uterine cancer. We've spent entire days together while she gets her chemo infusion, and I see how much care and love she gives to and receives from the staff. It's palpable, you can feel it.

My first husband had multi-visceral transplant surgery where they gave him a new liver, pancreas, stomach, and small intestine. He had a blood disorder that caused him to over-clot, thus the transplant came as a block of organs to include all the veins and arteries between the four organs. I spent most of a year with him in the hospital as his advocate, seeing firsthand the care and compassion from the surgeons, doctors, and nursing staff. So, believe me, I know how necessary these people are.

My point is that—sometimes—there may be another way. A different way. A way that doesn't involve seeing another specialist or taking yet another prescription medication. As you read along you will quickly see that I prefer, embrace, and advocate for a holistic approach to wellness.

Let me paint a picture. For over thirty years I worked in a private nonprofit Jesuit institute for higher education. The one word that truly matters in that sentence is "Jesuit." There is a Jesuit philosophy called *cura personalis*, which loosely translates to "care of the whole person." We don't just focus on academics and what happens in the classroom. We also care for the student's life experience on campus, whether he or she is a resident or commuter. We provide services that focus on physical activity, career guidance, social activities, organizations and clubs, spirituality, counseling, dining and food choices, internships, and community service, among other things. What we nurture goes beyond the "intellect of the head."

In the same way, I believe health-care professionals must care for more than just the body. We must care for the entire person as a whole entity. The human body is an integrated system; it's not separate body parts and organs held together with skin. Everything is interconnected. So how can we just treat one part? We must treat the entire system.

That entire system, the body, how it works, does not function in a bubble on its own. It has the air that we breathe, the environment around us, Mother Earth, and the miracles of nature. There is a universal spiritual harmony, and everything needs to work in sync for health to flourish. I'm here to tell you that the body, mind, and soul are driven, even preprogrammed, to work in harmony and because of this anything is possible. If we start to take matters into our own hands and treat our body like the temple it was created to be—naturally, holistically, toxic-free as it was originally designed—then we can live a life of optimal health. It is achievable, it is attainable!

Remember, there is no magic pill though. If you choose to embark on this journey, you may have a huge uphill battle on your hands. You may have to go against advice of those you hold dear. You may have to stand alone. This will take a lot of effort and dedication and time. In the end, however, it is worth it, because you will find, as I have, a loving and supportive group of people on a mission to heal the world. You will find you feel incredible, inspired, healthy, motivated, and eternally grateful. What better feeling is that? Doesn't that bring a smile to your face? Isn't that far better than the psychological fear induced by the experiment of thinking you are terminal or doomed to a life of illness and death?

I actively work to live an extraordinary life, and it has kept me 100% healthy. I mean it. My group of newly formed friends, professionals, collaborators all work toward health and extraordinary lives. But, it is not enough for me to simply be healthy. It is not enough to simply be disease free. My passion is to share how I have done it, how others have done it. By sharing leading research and studies, my goal is to ultimately walk you back to health. Isn't it time you learned that it truly is as Dr. Richard Schulze says: "Getting well is easy. It's getting sick that takes years of dedicated hard work." Isn't it time you learned how true this is and take action to change it?

My point, and in the end the reason for this book ... I want you to one day be able to tell me that you found your health easily and as a result you found your extraordinary!

PART ONE
Epigenetics

Chapter 1

Genetics, Epigenetics: What Do These Words Even Mean?

If genetics really isn't everything, as my title proposes, what does it mean to you and your possibly incurable or chronic or even unknown disease? As promised, I'm going to show you how you can not only get your "genes" to fit you, but you can reinforce the environment around you to do just that and more. Who wants to burst out of their jeans after all? Yes, a purposeful play on words. If you are bursting out of your jeans, you are denying your genetic body the help of reinforcing healing techniques that exist around you. I want us to be healthy, strong, fit, happy, and pursuing our true callings in life: not bursting out all over the place with bad behaviors, misdirection, lack of motivation, or lack of energy. I want to encourage everyone to take the small steps needed to modify your lifestyle, live a wonderful life, and let go of all the behaviors forcing you closer and closer to illness or even worse, death. For this reason I am sharing the stories of women who have taken matters into their own hands and given their genetic makeup a boost. As a result they are now healthy.

So, how do we go about making these changes, and why is it that we really do have a fighting chance to attain ultimate health despite what the medical community may make us believe?

Let us begin with science. Epigenetics, and for that matter, even genetics, are big words, so what exactly do they mean? The way most people think of genetics is as the material that makes up the DNA we have inherited biologically from our family through the ages. You hear a lot about this today on TV as people talk about things like ancestry and wanting to learn where they came from genetically, their ethnicity, their heritage. We also hear more and more about genetics and finding possible gene-specific links to cancer. These are general uses of the word *genetics* and mean that we are biologically analyzing the blueprint with which we are born—in other words, our "genetic" makeup or foundation.

For decades the medical establishment has believed the only thing that determines our future health is the genes we were born with. This has led to devoting billions of dollars to further research. Luckily the genetic theory alone, with scientific evidence to back it up, is expanding and people are becoming enlightened to the idea that genetics isn't everything. This expanded thinking is what triggered adding the prefix epi- (the three letters placed before the word *genetics*, which comes from the Greek language and means "on" or "upon") and has given scientists new theories to investigate. So, although epigenetics was loosely used in the early stages meaning "development that happens to the genes because of something going on around," like in the environment, it became an actual field of study starting in 1942 when Conrad H. Waddington coined the term.[1]

For those who need a little more background, the word *epigenesis* translated from Greek simply means "extra growth." If we take the concept that there are the genes that we are born with, and then there are the genes that have a possibility of being acted upon due to environment and sustenance and those that can actually grow stronger with proper care, we start to see that genetics isn't everything. This is exciting. This is inspiring because this tells us that we don't have to suffer the illnesses of our parents and grandparents that we were taught to believe we would have to endure as we age.

It is exciting to know that we have some control over our health destinies, and that if we start now we can stay healthy or get healthy and live wonderful lives into our 90s and even 100s. We can even avoid or rid ourselves of diabetes, obesity, and some arthritic disorders. Now, what pharmaceutical or medical team wants you to know that? This is why understanding the field of epigenetics is so important.

The true analysis of how our development and the environment impact our genes has only evolved in the last 10–15 years. You hear the term epigenetics more often and now people are even talking about epigenomics, in reference to the financial impact of epigenetics. But what matters to us mostly is getting to the heart of what that "on" or "upon" means and what we can do to help our genes so as to not get an illness.

---

1   "Epigenetics: Fundamentals – What Is Epigenetics?" http://www.whatisepigenetics. com/fundamentals/ (accessed March 8, 2017).

In an article entitled "6 Ways to Switch on Your Healthy, Happy Genes" by Dr. Roizen and Dr. Oz, whom most people have heard of, they explain epigenetics as "your epic ability to assert control over your DNA by switching certain genes on and silencing others. While you can't change your basic genetic code (DNA), you can make the best of what you have by changing your gene expression, or what gets turned on and what gets turned off."[2] The doctors go on to explain that "This new science is getting plenty of attention in the media, with headlines like 'Reprogram Your Genes' and 'How to Hack Your Own DNA,' and in scientific journals, too. There have been more than 10,000 research papers on epigenetics published in the past 10 years."[3]

This is an exciting field because with these discoveries comes more hope that we can allay illness and perhaps even slow down the aging process. What healthy person wouldn't want to live a longer life, after all?

When you think about it, the truth is, the average person knows very little about genes, DNA, chromosomes, mutations, and what medical doctors define as genetic illnesses. I want to begin by talking about original theories and genetics, more according to the layman because I am not a biologist, geneticist, or scientist. With the terms *genetics* and *epigenetics* so loosely thrown around with these discoveries, I want to address the way that I am using and defining the terms in the book, which is all about realizing that we do have control over our bodies and our genes and that we can make them stronger

---

2   "6 Ways to Switch on Your Healthy, Happy Genes," *AZ Daily Star*, February 16, 2015.
3   Ibid.

by building on the core, the DNA we were born with. Call it a small degree of creative license to prove my point—that even you can change and adapt and make whatever you were born with stronger ... better ...

Technically diseases like sickle-cell anemia, hemophilia, Down's syndrome, Huntington's disease, cystic fibrosis, and others are genetic diseases as defined by the medical community. If you are talking about a genetic disorder, you are normally talking about the mutation in the single base in the deoxyribonucleic acid, or DNA. "In the early 1950s two scientists, Rosalind Franklin and Maurice Wilkins, studied DNA using X-rays. Franklin produced an X-ray photograph that allowed two other researchers, James Watson and Francis Crick to work out the 3D structure of DNA. The structure of DNA was found to be a double helix."[4]

As research evolved it was discovered that our DNA is a pair (thus double helix) of 23 chromosomes. "Every person has two copies of each gene, one inherited from each parent. Most genes are the same in all people, except for a small number of genes (less than 1 percent of the total), which are slightly different between people."[5] In humans, each cell normally contains 23 pairs of chromosomes, for a total of 46. Twenty-two of these pairs, called autosomes, look the same in both males and females. The 23rd pair, the sex chromosomes, differ between males and females. Females have two copies of the X chromosome, while males have one X and one Y chromosome.[6]

---

4   "BBC – GCSE Bitesize: The Discovery of DNA." *Bbc.co.uk* http://www.bbc.co.uk/schools/gcsebitesize/science/add_edexcel/cells/dnarev3.shtml (accessed April 18, 2017).

5   Genetics. "What Is A Gene?." *Genetics Home Reference.* https://ghr.nlm.nih.gov/primer/basics/gene (accessed March 10, 2017).

6   Genetics. "How Many Chromosomes Do People Have?" *Genetics Home Reference.* https://ghr.nlm.nih.gov/chromosome/6 (accessed March 10, 2017).

Therefore when I am speaking of the "core" or the genetics we are born with, I am referring to the 46 chromosomes. But, what happens when a gene mutates? Think of it this way: "A gene mutation is a permanent alteration in the DNA sequence that makes up a gene, such that the sequence differs from what is found in most people. Mutations range in size; they can affect anywhere from a single DNA building block (base pair) to a large segment of a chromosome that includes multiple genes."[7]

Now, this is where it gets interesting. According to genetics today, there are two reasons for a gene mutating: one is hereditary and the other is acquired. "Hereditary mutations are inherited from a parent and are present throughout a person's life in virtually every cell in the body. These mutations are also called germline mutations because they are present in the parent's egg or sperm cells, which are also called germ cells. When an egg and a sperm cell unite, the resulting fertilized egg cell receives DNA from both parents. If this DNA has a mutation, the child that grows from the fertilized egg will have the mutation in each of his or her cells."[8] Simplified, if a person is born with a mutation from conception, it has been passed on through birth and is called a hereditary mutation. Remember, this is in *each* of the cells.

The second form of mutation is called an acquired mutation. "Acquired (or somatic) mutations occur at some time during a person's life and are present only in certain cells, not

7   Genetics. "What Is a Gene Mutation and How Do Mutations Occur?" *Genetics Home Reference.* https://ghr.nlm.nih.gov/primer/mutationsanddisorders/genemutation (accessed March 10, 2017).
8   Ibid.

in every cell in the body. These changes can be caused by environmental factors such as ultraviolet radiation from the sun, or can occur if a mistake is made as DNA copies itself during cell division. Acquired mutations in somatic cells (cells other than sperm and egg cells) cannot be passed on to the next generation."[9] Simplified, these are cells that mutate after birth and are not in every cell in the body. They can mutate due to the environment or some other factor that causes the cells to make a mistake in copying themselves when dividing. Again, this mistake happens to the individual only and is not passed on to future generations. There is supposedly no telling what will trigger this change or when.

What we are going to be addressing for the most part are the acquired or somatic mutations because those are the ones we can "save," "protect," and "enforce" so negative mutations don't occur. Our goal is to support our genes so we can remain healthy and live a long life. It is a process of taking the environmental factors, food factors, physical, emotional, and spiritual factors that affect us and strengthen our immune systems and bodies so that we can support whatever it is we were born with.

Since genetic inheritance is technically four-fold, there is the single gene inheritance as we discussed above, and then there is something called multifactoral inheritance that you can argue includes arthritis, diabetes, high blood pressure, heart disease, Alzheimer's disease, cancer, and obesity. This is where many factors influence what conditions the person has, or as some say, "inherits." There are heated debates that

---

9   Ibid.

continue today when it comes to genetics, and there are still physicians out there who say epigenetics is a scam because no environmental factor could possibly harm a person or mutate a gene. They are the ones who feel you can't avoid getting the illnesses your parents so kindly passed on to you.

Since I do not subscribe to that theory, I want to share one final bit of science. We've discussed the chromosomes and how they can mutate; now there are the energy-producing cells that I want to briefly discuss called mitochondria. "Mitochondria are structures within cells that convert the energy from food into a form that cells can use. Although most DNA is packaged in chromosomes within the nucleus, mitochondria also have a small amount of their own DNA (known as mitochondrial DNA or mtDNA). In some cases, inherited changes in mitochondrial DNA can cause problems with growth, development, and function of the body's systems. These mutations disrupt the mitochondria's ability to generate energy efficiently for the cell."[10] It is my belief that as we learn more about epigenetics, we will learn that if our energy structure has been impacted negatively by the environment, processed foods, toxins, bad air, bad water, plastics, negative thinking, depression, and the list goes on, it is here that we start to lose our footing with health. It is here that we need to, but more importantly have the power to, change—to reinforce so we can help our genes work more efficiently and keep the energy moving that we need not only to survive but to attain and remain in optimal health.

---

10   Genetics. "Can Changes in Mitochondrial DNA Affect Health and Development?" *Genetics Home Reference.* https://ghr.nlm.nih.gov/primer/mutationsanddisorders/mitochondrialconditions (accessed March 10, 2017).

At the end of the day we want our cells to generate energy efficiently and our mitochondria to function perfectly. We want every cell to be rejuvenated and healthy because then we are healthy ourselves. We have energy and can do the things we want to do to flourish and enjoy life as humans.

I am arming you with a small foundation of knowledge, again leaving the technical information to the scientists and pros. If this information is too technical, let it go, but on a personal note, I wanted to share because what I learned about this entire concept and field was so extraordinary that it propelled me to write a book.

When I came up with the idea and started the process of interviewing people who had beaten the odds and overcome their illnesses, the title *Genetics Isn't Everything* popped into my head. It came from my story, from me not getting all the diseases and conditions that seem to run rampant on both sides of my family tree.

At the time that my gut told me I needed to write about this, I did not have more than a basic understanding of genetics, but since I was in training to become a holistic health coach I was introduced to the word *epigenetics*. It started with a fascination from hearing Deepak Chopra say the following in a lecture that explored the concepts of universal consciousness and total well-being:

> Epigenetics is a new science. And it says that even though the sequence of your DNA may be fixed, how you turn on your genes and turn off the genes depends on the quality of your awareness. So, your thoughts,

your feelings, your emotions, your speech, your language, the way you use language, your personal relationships, your social interactions, of course your food, and the quality of your sleep. All these things influence the way our genes are regulated.[11]

Thinking about this, something resonated in me on a deeper level. How fascinating is it that our thoughts, emotions, and interactions can influence the way our genes are regulated? That is powerful because there are a lot of negative and fearful people out there. I have an analytical mind and a curious spirit, and this hypothesis started my journey to learn more, research more, interview more, and then share more. This blossomed into what has become the reason for this book and my purpose.

It started to dawn on me as I researched more on epigenetics that what happens to us is not strictly an outcome of our DNA. Initially the way I understood it is that our DNA is a blueprint of possible outcomes and that our environment, stress, food, etc., turn things on and/or off. So for example, if I had a lot more chronic stress in my life and ate horribly, like processed foods, etc., I probably would be right alongside my mom right now getting radiation and chemo for cancer or I would have had a heart attack in my forties like my dad and his brother. I've been able to avoid the cancer on my mom's side and the heart-related issues and obesity on my dad's side by being aware, making different lifestyle choices, and taking care of myself. This made me think that we are not just

---

11   "The Future of Well-Being with Deepak Chopra, MD; Deepak Chopra, MD, explores the concepts of universal consciousness and total well-being." Module 39 of the Health Coach Training Program at the Institute for Integrative Nutrition, Minute 17.

pawns sitting back waiting for what diagnosis the doctor one day gives us, but we are and can be proactive warriors who build up our defenses around us so no "gene" can stop us from health and living a wonderful and happy life—albeit sometimes with restrictions but those that are truly for our own good. We will not allow our precious bodies to be vulnerable because we have already reinforced them to preempt difficult environments. That's a revelation!

When we have moved into an age where most of the American population is obese and we can't fit into our "jeans," you know that it is time to start listening to what our true genes need and find ways to support them and protect them. We have moved into an age where information is everywhere and easily accessible, but why are we not listening? Why are we not learning? We walk around in distress looking to doctors for answers when the real answers are within us and around us, and believe it or not if we moved back to a simpler life and the core vegetation and hunting that was created at the beginning of time, like non-genetically-modified organic vegetables and fruits, antibiotic-free pasture-raised grass-fed animals, and wild caught fish, etc., we would all start to regain health. We would all begin to fit into our jeans and we would all be living healthier lives. What good is it to understand genetics and DNA sequencing if we have no intention of learning from it, seeing the harm that we are doing to ourselves, and putting our knowledge to good use to get healthy despite what certain industries say?

It's great to make a claim and realize that genetics isn't everything, that you do have control, that you don't have to accept illness and malaise as a way of life, and that you too can control your destiny. The question is, will you? Will you get proactive, will you make changes for yourself and your loved ones, and in turn will you share this with others? It is my intent to help educate my readers. To hopefully have you pick a story that resonates with you or a family member or friend so strongly that this catapults you to start to make changes and realize that there are others before you that have been there and conquered it.

Let's all become *"epic* geneticists" and bring in those warrior actions, those new and healthy habits that will strengthen our immune systems, eradicate our diseases, and let's spread the knowledge that we can all care more for the environment, our animals, and our bodies. We need to stop destroying things around us and start building healthier foundations. Now, wouldn't that be a life worth living and a purpose worthy of sharing?

Chapter 2

What Happens to Us Is *NOT* Strictly a Result of DNA

Your genome is like a giant never-ending piece of clay you can shape into whatever you want it to be.

*—Jason Shon Bennett,
HealthGuard Wellness*

Let's dive in and talk statistics. According to the CDC about 3–6% of children worldwide are born with serious birth defects every year.[12] That leaves 94–97% of the population born healthy. So, why is it today that over 90% of the population complains of feeling sick and tired on a regular basis? Why is it that despite being born healthy we now have so much cancer, heart disease, diabetes, obesity, and chronic illness? Is this not a glaring sign that we are actively doing something to make ourselves sick? What is the role of genetics

---

12   "World Birth Defects Day." Centers for Disease Control and Prevention. https://www.cdc.gov/features/birth-defects-day/ (accessed March 10, 2017).

and epigenetics in medical conditions then, and do we have control over our genes?

According to *Statistics at a Glance: The Burden of Cancer in the United States*, "Approximately 39.6 percent of men and women will be diagnosed with cancer at some point during their lifetimes (based on 2010–2012 data)."[13] According to *Statistics at a Glance: The Burden of Cancer Worldwide*, "Cancer is among the leading causes of death worldwide. In 2012, there were 14 million new cases and 8.2 million cancer-related deaths worldwide."

According to the National Center of Health Statistics, the leading causes of death in the United States in 2016 were: Heart disease: 614,348, Cancer: 591,699, Chronic lower respiratory diseases: 147,101, Accidents (unintentional injuries): 136,053, Stroke (cerebrovascular diseases): 133,103, Alzheimer's disease: 93,541, Diabetes: 76,488, Influenza and pneumonia: 55,227, Nephritis, nephrotic syndrome, and nephrosis: 48,146, Intentional self-harm (suicide): 42,773.[14]

That is a lot of heart disease, cancer, and chronic lower respiratory illnesses taking the lives of our loved ones. The statistics in America are just plain frightening. What I find even more shocking is a recent article I came upon that the average American is dying earlier now versus living longer. How scary is that?

In an article in *The Atlantic Daily* it stated, "For the first time since the 1990s, Americans are dying at a faster rate, and

---

13   "Cancer Statistics." *National Cancer Institute*. https://www.cancer.gov/about-cancer/ understanding/statistics (accessed March 10, 2017).

14   "Faststats." 2017. *Cdc.Gov*. https://www.cdc.gov/nchs/fastats/leading-causes-of-death. htm (accessed May 8, 2017).

they're dying younger. A pair of new studies suggest Americans are sicker than people in other rich countries, and in some states, progress on stemming the tide of basic diseases like diabetes has stalled or even reversed. The studies suggest so-called 'despair deaths'—alcoholism, drugs, and suicide—are a big part of the problem, but so is obesity, poverty, and social isolation."[15] As you will note, each one of these deaths could be ceased with intervention. The article went on to discuss the highest deaths and statistics confirming the National Center of Health Statistics rates above. This means that if people realized the fate of their genes and their lives could be partially taken into their own hands, then millions of lives per year could be saved. Epigenetics.

Now, to add to the fear factor of what we are doing to ourselves and our children, another fascinating but sad statistic about birth defects is that "About 10 percent of problems seen at birth can be traced to a specific agent (environmental agent, drug, biologic, or nutritional factor). About 20 percent are inherited or are associated with chromosomal changes. The rest (about 70 percent) are of unknown etiology, although a 1991 report from the General Accounting Office found that a majority of experts believe that a quarter or more of birth defects will be found to have been environmentally induced."[16]

So, let me clarify for you: if a quarter or more of birth defects are environmentally induced, if a major proportion of cancers are due to environmental toxins and not genetic

---

15   2017. https://www.theatlantic.com/health/archive/2016/12/why-are-so-many-ameri-cans-dying-young/510455/ (accessed May 8, 2017).

16   "Birth Defect Statistics." 2017. *The Physicians Committee.* http://www.pcrm.org/re-search/resch/reschethics/birth-defect-statistics (accessed March 10, 2017).

defects, if things like heart disease, diabetes, lung and liver illnesses were taken off the table because we controlled what we put in our mouths, on our skin, and we removed all forms of toxins from our environment, we would thereby remove all but about 20% (or less) of early deaths, leaving those to accident, actual old age, and suicide. I would even go as far as saying that many suicides would be prevented because some of the agents causing mental illness would no longer affect a person psychologically, or I would at least propose that a person who is happy and pain free is less likely to want to take their own life.

In discovering how bad the statistics are, it confirmed to me the question of how far do we have to go, how much worse do we have to be, to make change? Think about it: is a lifestyle change really that bad? That difficult? When does it become worth it?

I mean, how many times do you get together with friends and family and all they talk about is their aches and pains, and oh, this medicine and that problem—it's hard to stay positive in a world where there is so much physical and emotional pain. Yet, what are we doing to stop it? Is that fabricated food, that chemical soda really worth your life?

Aren't the statistics horrifying enough from a few years ago that 1 out of 3 women are going to die of cancer? Think of three of your closest female friends; now think of one of them gone. Yup, it's that simple if we don't start making change now. According to the above statistics, almost 1 out of every 2 of us will have some form of cancer! Is this okay? We need to be shocked into reality with these numbers.

I came upon an article that I want to share because it confirms everything I have been thinking and was eye-opening enough I wanted to share most of it. It was an article in *The Observer* (Gladstone, Australia) on October 6, 2016 called "Lifestyle Wins over Genetics; Our Healthy Choices Have Huge Impact" that explains so much. It starts by sharing that it has been "proven through the genetic study called The Genome Project, each one of your genes can create up to 30,000 proteins, any and all of which can create a different outcome—you get sick or you stay healthy. The aspects that activate or suppress your genes are almost always lifestyle-related. Your genome is like a giant never-ending piece of clay you can shape into whatever you want it to be."[17]

Cardiologist Dr. John Day said in 2014: "Most people think it's their genes, but the research on 3000 identical twins showed 25% of their longevity was due to genes. The other 75% was lifestyle."[18] This is fascinating, and I even share a story in this book on twins.

Dan Beuttner, in *The Blue Zones*, said: "Contrary to popular opinion, genes dictate as little as 2% of our life expectancy."

The 100-year genetic study by the University of Gothenburg found: "Hereditary factors don't play a major role. Lifestyle has the biggest impact. We do not inherit mortality to any great extent, but instead it is the sum of our own habits that has the biggest impact."

---

17 "Lifestyle Wins over Genetics; Our Healthy Choices Have Huge Impact," The Observer (Gladstone, Australia), October 6, 2016.
18 Ibid.

Yes, your genes have an influence on your health and longevity, but the trick is that they are triggered by you and your diet and lifestyle.

Your health is the cumulative experience of your lifetime.

You have the power to change it with every mouthful.

A healthy, plant-based whole-food diet gives you healthy genetic expression in the gut.

Groundbreaking 2014 research by Cardiff University School of Medicine from The Caerphilly Cohort Study tracked the diet and lifestyle choices made by a group of men for 35 years, from 1979 to 2014.

"In 1979, about 2500 men were advised to make healthy choices. Only 25 of them succeeded in actually doing it."[19] My book inadvertently became all about women, but I can assure you that we are often no better about taking matters into our own hands. Perhaps those who care and nurture their children may increase the odds of actually succeeding at making healthier choices, but a huge part of our problem today is that we have so many options and feel so entitled to use and abuse the options that we are actually shortening our own life spans.

According to the article, "These men lived significantly longer than men who did not follow the recommended diet and lifestyle steps, with disease hitting them at much older ages.

The researchers found the men who followed the advice had: 70% lower rates of diabetes, 60% lower rates of heart

---

19   Ibid.

attack, 60% lower rates of stroke, 60% lower rates of dementia, and 40% lower rates of cancer.

These incredible results, in real time, on real people, regardless of their genetics or hereditary health issues, are far more powerful than any drug or medication ever invented. Those who did none of the five strategies 'experienced no health benefit at all.'

What were the five recommended steps the men took?

A healthy, balanced, whole-food diet;

Regular daily exercise;

Maintaining a healthy weight;

Low or no alcohol consumption; and,

Not smoking.

You own your genetics so make them work for you!

Everyone is different and each person's genes have a particular influence. However, here is the real kicker: you have the genes you have and the only thing you can control is the environment they live in and how they are expressed."[20]

Right? Exactly as stated above, "You own your genetics so make them work for you!" This article has expressed my points exactly. In the end my goal is to not let you—or me for that

---

20 Ibid.

matter—be a statistic. It is for me to help you pull up all those warrior actions that can come in to help protect us and take back our health. We can only blame our DNA so far, we can only blame our possible inherited illnesses so far, and then we need to take action. As the above article states, "Your genome is like a giant never-ending piece of clay you can shape into whatever you want it to be." To me that is empowering.

Is this not a glaring sign that we are actively doing something to make ourselves sick? In opposition, isn't this a sign that we can actually grab control over our genes—genome, as the quote says—work it like clay, and shape it into anything you want it to be?

And how liberating to know as the Gothenberg study above states, "We do not inherit mortality to any great extent, but instead it is the sum of our own habits that has the biggest impact." Well, that is to those of us willing to take action and become accountable for what we put in and on our skin! I assure you that the women who share their journeys in this book will prove just that.

The article ends with the same thought I want to leave you with ... "Even the near-40-year-old Okinawa Centenarian Study has confirmed diet and lifestyle are what create the healthiest and longest-living centenarians—not genetics, good luck or good genes."[21] So, what are we collectively going to do about that?

---

21   Ibid.

Chapter 3

Genetic Makeup: How S.A.D. Our Standard American Diet Is Killing Us

Fast food is popular because it's convenient, it's cheap, and it tastes good. But the real cost of eating fast food never appears on the menu.

—Eric Schlosser

When you read the journeys in this book, you are going to start to see some common threads. There are people who were so sick they knew they either had to follow doctors' orders with little hope and fewer answers or take matters into their own hands. Many were so ill that they could barely function, but some last bit of super-human energy or an epiphany hit them, forcing changes they knew they probably should have triggered but had not gotten around to—changes that surprisingly transformed their lives. Considering the years of cumulative damage for some, their healing came relatively quickly—on the scale of things. Some were told they would live with this chronic condition forever … but you'll be glad to learn they worked their way to health.

Over the course of my lifetime, with the help of these stories and my various studies, I've learned that there are four main areas of our lifestyle that can fortify, that strengthen, the genes we were born with and in a sense work as protective cover-up for our bodies. These four areas are our diet, mindset, physical activity, and environment. I'll cover each of these in this chapter.

Think about what many women do every morning as they put on makeup. Where do they start after they wash their face? They take the next step and put on "foundation." A word that was created because every piece of makeup put on over the foundation will last longer, and it creates the base so the overall process works better. Now imagine if unknowingly you start by washing your face in chlorine and fluoride, use Vaseline or petroleum-based products as a foundation, and then move on to place carcinogenic fillers to erase wrinkles. Do you really think we are doing our body or even our face any long-term favors? No, chances are we are starting our day helping our body become toxic.

Now think of your day starting out with the purest of ingredients, a healthy foundation—one our whole body and skin can love. That is the picture of radiance I want you to embrace. It is the piece where we protect our organs, and it certainly doesn't mean starting the next "nutritional" and nourishing step of our day killing ourselves with our Standard American

Diet (SAD), which is low in fiber and plant-based foods and high in processed foods and animal fats.

I confirmed for myself, and now for you, through these stories and with my studies to become a certified health coach from the highly respected Institute for Integrative Nutrition (IIN) that wellness is not only about nutrition. It's much more than what you put on your plate and into your body. It's a combination of everything that makes up your particular lifestyle, including things like your physical activities, spirituality, career, personal and professional relationships and interactions, continuing education, financial situation, where you live geographically, your home life, etc. Think of it like this: if you have a wonderful loving relationship with your partner, are in good health, love your job, find comfort in your spiritual practice, but are struggling financially—then you are not well. Financial struggles bring stress and worry into your daily life, which in turn affects your overall health and wellness.

Here's another example. A single woman living alone comes home from work at the end of the day and binges on everything in her cupboards and freezer. If that woman came home to a partner or even a roommate, it's less likely she would binge. Having a loving relationship fills a void that food cannot. Life is about balance, and if something is out of balance it will eventually impact your health.

In my introduction, I stated that I'm sharing stories about people who have changed their health and thus their lives with nutrition, self-care, and self-compassion. In this instance, nutrition does in fact mean nutrition, as it is a crucial factor for optimal health. What I focus on and recommend to my clients are organic, local, and seasonal foods. Organic is critical since non-organic fruits and vegetables are inundated with pesticides, which wreak havoc on our body's internal systems. In terms of animal proteins, organic means they have not been infused with antibiotics, steroids, and growth hormones, which you would be ingesting by default.

Local foods are always best, because they don't have to travel very far to get to you. If you are eating fruits from South America, for instance, they were picked long before they were ripe and then end up ripening, somewhat, on the refrigerated vehicle on which they were transported. Thus, they were picked off the vine before fully ripe, meaning they didn't have enough time to absorb all the nutrients from the soil that they should have. Because they haven't been able to ripen in their natural environment, fruits and vegetables that have to be transported long distances also don't develop their natural full flavor.

Eat what's in season. There are many reasons for this, one being it's cheaper because it's more abundant in your geographical location. It doesn't have to be shipped from anywhere, saving transportation costs. It also supports your local community. What's in season is more flavorful as it's fresher. Additionally, when you eat what's in season, you have variety all year long. There is also a macrobiotic principle, which focuses on creating a yin-yang balance in all things in life, such as within your body as well as your environment. When you eat local foods in season, you are in harmony with nature.[22]

22 "Is Your Body Begging You to Go Macrobiotic?" 2017. Dr. Axe. https://draxe.com/macrobiotic-diet/ (accessed April 22, 2017).

What I've just described here is not the Standard American Diet, which is SAD in more ways than one. Pun intended. The typical diet in this country is loaded with bad fats, conventional animal proteins, sugar and other artificial sweeteners, alcohol, GMO-laden grains, and packaged chemicalized food-products. (I can't in good faith call these things food.) To add insult to injury, most packaged food-products in this country are loaded with high-fructose corn syrup, or something very similar with new names that constantly crop up to fool us into thinking it's healthy.

I'm generalizing, of course, but most Americans do not eat enough fruits and vegetables, and when we do, they are loaded with chemical fertilizers and pesticides, which I cover a little later. We also consume too many bad fats such as hydrogenated oils made from corn, peanut, and soybeans, and other genetically modified cooking oils. If you want to be healthier, change your fats to extra-virgin olive oil, coconut oil, and grass-fed butter or ghee. Eat avocados! They are chock-full of healthy fats and have loads of fiber—another macronutrient largely missing in Americans.

Sadly, most Americans are always in a rush and choose convenience and speed over healthfulness. Think drive-thrus and fast food. We as a nation are not getting enough vitamins, essential nutrients, minerals, plant-based foods, and good fats.[23] We need to pay attention to what goes in our mouths and remember, even the smallest steps will help your body heal.

23 "9 Charts That Show The Standard American Diet." 2017. *Dr. Axe.* https://draxe.com/charts-american-diet (accessed April 23, 2017).

Earlier, I mentioned self-care and self-compassion. To me, self-care means time to yourself, by yourself, and for yourself—in whatever way works for you and your particular lifestyle. It could be a monthly massage, a walk at lunchtime, taking time to read for fun or for personal growth, or a nightly bath; it's time alone just for you on a regular basis.

We all have many, many things to handle in any given day. Spouse, kids, career, school, aging parents, groceries, laundry, housekeeping—you get the picture. So how do we fit it all in? How do we make sure we can fit it all in? For me, personally, I let housekeeping fall to the bottom of the list. I'll get to it when I get to it. It's just not that important. What is important is to plan time into your day to take care of you. Actually schedule "me-time" into your calendar or to-do list. In a way that's meaningful for you. This is not selfish! It's an absolute must.

Perhaps it's an early-morning run before the kids get up, or closing your office door and doing yoga for 30 minutes (if you're lucky enough to have an office door). Taking a walk in the middle of the day. Reading on the train—something *not work-related*. Writing in a journal. Writing a blog. Meditation, exercise, alone time, bourbon, fine wine—the list is endless. Bottom line: you must take care of your body, your mind, and your spirit. These mean different things to different people, so you need to figure out what this means for you. Then do it.

When and if someone in your family needs you, you want to be able to help. That can only happen if you are well. That can only happen if you take care of yourself first.

Self-compassion is a bit different, and while I have some expertise as my PhD dissertation was focused on compassion, the best definition I've seen for self-compassion was from Dr. Kristen Neff, founder of self-compassion.org. Dr. Neff defined self-compassion as having three elements: mindfulness, self-kindness, and connectedness.[24] Mindfulness is a lot like being present in the moment. It's about recognizing what's going on inside you, in a nonjudgmental way. If you are having negative thoughts, for example, observe and take note of what's happening without overreacting and without trying to ignore or suppress them. Acknowledge and accept the thoughts.

Dr. Neff describes self-kindness as being supportive and kind to ourselves instead of being "harshly self-critical." When you feel inadequate or you've made a mistake, take a step back and realize that like every other human being—we are not perfect. So, be gentle with yourself. Have the same sympathy for yourself as you would have towards others. This is a great segue to connectedness because it helps us remember that we are not alone. All humans suffer in one way or another; it's part of the "shared human experience." You will see all kinds of suffering as you dive deeper into this book. You are not alone.

Personally, I meditate, I eat healthy, I exercise, I take time to read, I take walks at lunch, I take detox salt baths, I get massages and pedicures, I go out into nature, I camp in the winter, and sometimes I play word games on my phone such as "WordBrain." I don't do all these things every day. I do what feels appropriate for the moment. But I take the time to do what I need for me. As should you.

---

24   Neff, Kristin, What Self-Compassion?, What Not, Tips practice, Videos Self-Compassion, and MSC Intensives et al. 2017. "Definition and Three Elements of Self-Compassion | Kristin Neff." *Self-Compassion.* http://self-compassion.org/the-three-elements-of-self-compassion-2/ (accessed April 22, 2017).

When it comes to exercise, the best advice I ever heard was to find something you love doing. If you enjoy it, then it never becomes something you *have* to do or *should* do. It's something you find fun and enjoyable, so you'll keep on doing it. In Jess's story you'll read that she thought back to the things she loved to do as a child. She also replaced the word *exercise* with *activity*. Now she does these activities with her children. She gets to see the joy on their faces as they do healthy activities together. It doesn't get any better than that.

The bottom line is that exercise doesn't have to be a chore, it doesn't have to be intense, and it doesn't have to be a marathon. It is something that is critical to your overall health and well-being, though, so don't ignore it. According to Dr. Mercola, exercise has many health benefits, such as better sleep, weight loss or gain, improved immunity, and improved brain function including memory.[25]

Another great piece of advice is to listen to your body. This is true in general, but also with exercise. Don't push past your current limits. If all you can manage is a five-minute walk, then only walk for five minutes. The next time you go out for a walk, try six. Never compete with anyone else as everyone has his or her own story. Only try to be better than who you were yesterday.

Yoga is an amazing way to improve your physical condition, core strength, and flexibility. It's also one of those types of conditioning that is easily modifiable so that you don't have to jump straight into a contorted position if you are less than flexible. There are blocks and straps and other tools available

---

25 "Exercise to Optimize Your Health – Mercola.Com." 2017. *Fitness.Mercola.Com* http://fitness.mercola.com/sites/fitness/exercises.aspx (accessed April 23, 2017).

to help ease you into the various poses—or as they are called in yoga, *asanas.*

Some people may associate yoga with stretching, which in a way it is, but it is also so much more than that. Back when I was doing yoga regularly, like four times per week, I remember it being the only time when the rest of the world disappeared. When I was taking a yoga class, the only thing on my mind was the particular pose I was doing at the moment. I wasn't wondering if I needed to stop at the grocery store or whether I had any clean underwear. I was completely focused on where I was in the present moment.

According to Dr. Weil, in India, yoga is considered an ancient science; "a philosophical-religious system for attaining unity of consciousness."[26] This is something on my to-do list; to get back into yoga and re-attain that unity of consciousness.

If you searched the Internet for exercise, you would find approximately 22 million results. Some of the recommendations might be to do an hour of exercise five days per week, while others say a half hour five days per week. Other sites will suggest more vigorous forms of exercise, and some are proponents of more gentle, centering ones. The truth is, exercise needs are as uniquely individualized as we humans are. Pick something you love, or try out a bunch of different types of exercise and rule out the ones you can't stand, but have fun doing it!

---

26 Wellness, Health, Balanced Living, and Exercise Fitness. 2017. "Yoga: More Than a Workout – Dr. Weil." Drweil.Com. https://www.drweil.com/health-wellness/balanced-living/exercise-fitness/yoga-more-than-a-workout/ (accessed April 23, 2017).

Now as we work to keep our body moving, well-oiled, and supple, we have to take time to explore and understand our precious environment and the harm we are doing with all the toxins we are using and spreading and the impact it has on our lives. There is so much to say on this topic I'm not even sure where to begin.... In current 21st-century time, we, the people of Earth, are bombarded with toxins on a daily basis. It's unavoidable. Besides the obvious, like air pollution and car exhaust, there's our water supply. If you are drinking water straight out of the tap—even in NY where it's supposedly the best—use a filter. Think I'm wrong? Read this: http://www.riverkeeper.org/campaigns/tapwater/is-my-tap-water-safe-to-drink-fact-sheet/. Those of you using well water aren't out of the woods either, as there is always the potential for soil contamination.

Okay, besides air pollution and tap water, what else is there? Well, if you aren't eating organic, you run the risk of ingesting pesticides, fungicides, and herbicides from fruits and vegetables as well as steroids, hormones, and antibiotics in animal proteins. There are toxins in our carpeting, sofas, mattresses where we spend one third of our lives, wood and laminate flooring, and dry cleaning. There are even toxins in our laundry detergent, dishwashing liquids, and household cleaning supplies. I won't even go into all the bad stuff that's in shampoos, conditioners, soaps, lotions, and cosmetics, except to say that our skin is the body's largest organ and it absorbs everything we put on it. Everything! Sadly, there is even published research that found "an average of 200 industrial compounds, pollutants, and other chemicals" in newborn babies.[27] Babies! Newborn babies!

By now you might be thinking, don't our bodies have internal filtering systems? Yes, they do. Our bodies are amazing pieces of machinery. They keep a steady temperature, they keep us breathing, they keep our hearts pumping, blood circulating, brain synapses firing, etc. They do all of this in split-seconds and all at the same time while we walk around and interact with other humans. Amazing! The human body's filtering method includes the liver, kidneys, lungs, spleen, lymphatic system, and skin.

However, due to all of the above, this constant assault day after day, month after month, year after year has caused our body's natural filters to become clogged. They are so clogged that they cannot keep up with the constant overload. The result is increased fat. Your body tries to protect itself and encapsulates toxins in your fat cells, so they can't harm other parts of your body. Ever wonder why you can't seem to lose those extra few pounds around your middle?[28]

What can we do? First, explore elimination diets because even the smallest removal of certain foods from your diet can help you heal. Some require you to avoid corn, soy, dairy, wheat, and gluten, and others have you avoid sugar, caffeine, and alcohol. No matter what, try your best to eat clean,

27 "Detailed Findings." 2017. *EWG*. http://www.ewg.org/research/body-burden-pollution-newborns/detailed-findings (accessed April 25, 2017).
28 "Toxins in Your Fat Cells Are Making You Sick and Bloated! Here's How You Can Cleanse Them! – David Avocado Wolfe." 2017. *David Avocado Wolfe*. https://www.davidwolfe.com/toxins-fat-cells-cleanse (accessed April 25, 2017).

organic, local, seasonal, whole foods in a rainbow of colors. If you eat animal proteins, stick with wild-caught fish, grass-fed beef, and pasture-raised poultry. Stay hydrated. I always recommend you drink half your body weight in ounces of water. So a 200-lb man should average 100 ounces of water per day. Add probiotics for good gut health. Replace white rice with brown rice or quinoa, which is higher in protein and fiber. Add nuts, beans, and legumes. Fruits, especially berries and avocados, are wonderful! It all comes back to diet. We all take showers every day to clean our outsides, why not pay attention to cleaning our insides?

These are just a few areas that we can begin to make slow but specific changes. All of these areas where we are supporting the genes we were born with fall under the realm of epigenetics. It's about the lifestyle choices you make on a daily basis. It all comes down to choice. When you choose ice cream over fruit for dessert, you are choosing sickness. When you choose forgiveness over anger, you are choosing wellness. When you choose to take a walk outside instead of sitting on the couch, you are choosing health.

Remember this: you get to choose. You get to choose whether to worry needlessly over something that will most likely never happen, or to let it go and trust that the Universe has your back. You get to choose how you feel. If you're in a bad mood for some reason, guess what? You can choose to change how you feel. Jump up and dance in your kitchen. Sing at the top of your lungs. Laugh at nothing. Then see how you feel. You get to choose. Always! When you choose something that brings you towards health, you win. And your jeans fit better.

Why? Because you supported, loved, and cared for the genes you were born with! No more SADness. A few small steps with whole foods and less toxic environments and I promise you will be headed towards healing and optimal health.

PART TWO

Thyroid And The Misdiagnosis Dilemma

In order to share the stories of women (sorry, men—it just happened this way; don't worry, I'm working on a book for you!) who have overcome a series of illnesses that many other people are struggling with today, I have broken this book into four major components related to specific illnesses that are plaguing our nation. Illnesses that are related to the thyroid, invisible illnesses like fibromyalgia and migraines, illnesses visible partially on the outside such as psoriasis and lupus, and illnesses that have a mental component such as eating disorders and depression.

After a general discussion of who is affected and what the illness or condition means, I share personal stories that show how people have succeeded in overcoming their conditions. Yes, I mean it: they healed their own illnesses!

Success stories play a vital role in our healing because the doom and gloom we are normally faced with when we are struggling with a physical illness become stories of hope. If others have done it, have found answers, have started or successfully healed themselves, then we can too.

I discuss each person's journey from four important areas: what they have endured, how they have healed, what inspiration they can provide—with tips for getting better—and finally how to contact them so if you or a loved one is struggling, you may reach out for help.

I have done the best I can to keep the stories simple and conversational because I want everyone to learn and understand what I am saying. By keeping it in this tone, my desire is that this will give you the strength to start one small, manageable step at a time. From there the possibilities will become endless! And, don't forget, all these women have made it their dream to help you heal—so don't hesitate one second to reach out and contact them. I send you healing and positive energy as you embark on a life of health and say good-bye to a life of illness.

Chapter 4

Thyroid: The Most Misdiagnosed Illness Today

Despite what most physicians may be willing to admit, more than 40%[29] of the female population in the United States suffers from a thyroid illness or disease. There is growing concern that not only are lab tests misread by physicians, but that there are a growing number of faulty ranges being disseminated. Regardless, I am not here to discuss the errors in the system, but rather to share stories of those who suffered from a problem involving their thyroid and found a way to heal by taking matters in their own hands.

As a visual experiment, the next time you are in a regular grocery or department store, take a look at the number of women who are losing their hair or have very thin hair on their scalps—that is, if they are not already wearing a wig or extensions. Do you think this is normal? Do you think this is healthy? We may be seeing this so often we feel it is normal, but I assure you, it is not. We are supposed to have healthy

---

29   "Hypothyroidism Diet + Natural Treatment – Dr. Axe." 2017. *Dr. Axe.* https://draxe.com/hypothyroidism-diet-natural-treatment/ (accessed April 4, 2017).

heads of hair, grow nails, and keep supple skin well into our 80s. Unfortunately, as a direct response to the unhealthy processed food and hormones found in the wrong places, like our drinking water, our eggs, and our meat, we are consuming and breathing toxins that are directly attacking our organs. We are a society that is slowly killing ourselves, and we just don't seem to want to pay attention.

Next time you are out in public, eavesdrop; listen to the number of people who complain of fatigue, who are gaining weight, losing hair and feel depressed, or perhaps even talk about feeling brain-fogged and exhausted. The situation is not getting better. It is moving into pandemic numbers, and the saddest part is that most women don't even realize that this is what they are suffering from. Some associate it with the normal process of aging, which by the way it is not, and some are already too tired to even try to find a solution because they are just fighting to get through the day.

Imagine, though, if we could walk up to everyone and educate them on what is happening. If we can share that there is a very real possibility their thyroid has been impacted from decisions they make in their daily lives, but that there is a chance to turn their situation and suffering around. Imagine being able to educate people enough to encourage them to search for more answers and learn about this incredible body of ours with a key organ called the thyroid. Imagine healing 40% of the population simply by learning what I learned below as a result of interviewing women who have suffered and yet have overcome. Even if you only take small bits of information from what I am about to share, you will have potentially learned more than some physicians are still being taught in their medical schools. Please, take what you can from this, and in your own time feel free to explore the resources I have shared so you can learn even more.

For those of you who don't know, the thyroid gland is a vital organ found in the neck—that beautiful butterfly-shaped organ below the Adam's apple. It is the regulator of metabolism because it converts oxygen and calories to energy. (Yes, women do have small Adam's apples, they are just not as visible and as large as men's.) When you go to your doctor's office and they put their fingers on your neck below the Adam's apple, they are touching to feel whether or not there is a lump or swelling to your thyroid. If there is a mass that the doctor can feel, it is most likely a goiter and you will be sent for more lab work and evaluations.

Here is where it gets tricky, though. If it can't be felt but you have a perceptive doctor who listens to you and can see the way you look (puffy skin and bags under eyes, swelling, weight gain, loss of hair, etc.) and listens to how you say you feel, they will know it is indicative of a thyroid problem and they will order lab work. Yes, a blood test. The physician normally looks at something called TSH, T3, and T4, but these results can be misleading because what the current field of endocrinology calls the "normal" range is what functional medical doctors who specialize in looking at the whole body and how it is functioning (versus just the thyroid) call the "sick" range.

But let us first start with a strange and fascinating genetic fact. Of all the genetic illnesses that infants are born with, according to the National Institute of Health (NIH), the likelihood of genetic hypothyroidism is very low and only about one out of every 4,000 newborns is actually born with a thyroid disorder.[30] Therefore, where is all this thyroid disease coming from? Even proposing that a person is "more likely to develop hypothyroidism if they have a close family member with an autoimmune disease,"[31] what makes 40% of the female population suffer? My point is that with such a small genetic impact to our population at birth, it is most definitely a case where epigenetic interventions can start to save us.

There is no doubt environment, food, toxins, and lifestyle all come into play. So how does this little organ work and what exactly damages or confuses it? The thyroid gland is an H-shaped organ composed of two lobes joined by a narrow isthmus located just below the laryngeal cartilages. The normal thyroid weighs approximately 15 to 25 g, with each lobe 4 to 6 cm in length and 1.3 to 1.8 cm in thickness.[32] It is a small organ but a powerful one. It is made up of small sacs and is filled with an iodine-rich protein called thyroglobulin along with the thyroid hormones thyroxine (T4) and small amounts of triiodothyronine (T3).[33]

The production of T4 and T3 in the thyroid gland is regulated by the hypothalamus and pituitary gland. To ensure stable levels of thyroid hormones, the hypothalamus monitors

30   Ibid.
31   Ibid.
32   "Thyroid Ultrasound." 2017. *Med-Ed.Virginia.Edu*. https://www.med-ed.virginia.edu/courses/rad/Thyroid_Ultrasound/01intro/intro-01-02.html (accessed April 5, 2017).
33   "Role of the Thyroid | Life Extension." 2017. *Lifeextension.Com*. http://www.lifeextension.com/Protocols/Metabolic-Health/Thyroid-Regulation/Page-02 (accessed January 22, 2017).

circulating thyroid hormone levels and responds to low levels by releasing thyrotropin-releasing hormone (TRH). This TRH then stimulates the pituitary to release thyroid-stimulating hormone (TSH).[9,10] When thyroid hormone levels increase, production of TSH decreases, which in turn slows the release of new hormone from the thyroid gland.[34] You need these hormones to metabolize food, to have energy, and to function—to say nothing about feeling fabulous.

This is a complicated process and I'm not expecting you to understand all of this, but I am hoping that if you can learn anything that you will start with the fact that the thyroid gland needs iodine and the amino acid L-tyrosine to make T4 and T3. A diet deficient in iodine can limit how much T4 the thyroid gland can produce and lead to hypothyroidism.[35]

It is interesting that we are told in the United States that a thyroid problem should not be a factor since cretinism was diagnosed decades ago and that the source of the problem was a mother deficient in iodine. Cretin children were being born severely mentally and physically stunted because their mother had a hypothyroid while the baby was conceived and growing in the womb. When it was discovered that cretin births decreased by giving moms iodine, the government decided that they should take measures into their own hands and now include iodine in our salt. While this might have been an altruistic step, and most certainly stopped many birth defects, it did not address why the moms were all lacking in iodine in the first place. To this day no government agency or medical

---

34   Ibid., 3.
35   Ibid.

establishment is saying that eating processed foods, being exposed to harmful toxins, an overuse of antibiotics and vaccines, etc., is the reason so many suffer from thyroid illnesses today.

Skip to 2017, where pregnancies are now monitored and moms' thyroids are pretty much checked as part of a wellness exam; why are there still so many women suffering? Why are men even showing more signs of a sick thyroid? Also, think of the health-conscious person who has gone to the opposite degree to never eat processed food and to abstain from salt other than healthy sea salt, and despite eating well still does not get enough of or even the type of iodine they need? What is it that we are missing to keep our thyroids functioning optimally?

To be honest, it is a little too early in the scientific stage to determine 100% of the reasons, but it will be a new and interesting hypothesis to study one day and learn all of the reasons our thyroids are being damaged. But, for now, there are two main diagnoses of thyroid disease, although subclinical sections fall within each, and that is hyper (overactive) or hypo (underactive) thyroid, with the latter being most common. Terms you might have heard are Hashimoto's for underactive thyroid and Graves' for overactive thyroid, but they are considered two sides of the same coin. Both present challenges. Just because you think you have been diagnosed with a hyperactive thyroid doesn't necessarily mean you will always have a symptom of losing weight!

In case you are interested in learning which range your thyroid falls in, remembering that I am not a doctor and can't give medical advice, should you have a blood test done there is a wonderful and holistic group known as Life Extension. They suggest an optimal level of TSH between 1.0 and 2.0 µIU/mL, as some studies have noted that a TSH above 2.0 may be associated with adverse cardiovascular risk factors.[26] In addition, a TSH between 1.0 and 2.0 µIU/mL has been associated with the lowest subsequent incidence of abnormal thyroid function.[66] However, while a measure of TSH alone is a useful screening tool in assessing thyroid function, Life Extension advocates additional testing, including Free T3 and T4 levels, to provide a more complete evaluation of the thyroid.[36] I recommend going to their site and reading more about the process, and you can even order a blood test through them if you are not getting the medical advice you feel you need. The site is http://www.lifeextension.com/vitamins-supplements/itemlc100018/comprehensive-thyroid-panel-blood-test and they have trained staff to walk you through the results. They will even collaborate with your doctor if you need them to.

In January 2017, Dr. Izabella Wentz did an amazing series on the thyroid called "The Thyroid Secret," and it revealed a number of people who have suffered misdiagnoses or poor medical recommendations, and it discussed how to treat yourself naturally. The stories, including her own, were incredible, and the participating patients and doctors were so much more knowledgeable than we find in the traditional medical community. Once again it started with a story of one person who suffered and who is coming forward with professional degrees and first-hand knowledge of what a thyroid disease took from her that

---

36   Ibid., 6.

launched into a worldwide awakening. It encourages people not to give up, because there is hope as you will see with the stories I share.

One particular episode discussed the importance of the gut. Most people don't think of the gut as something that can control the thyroid, but it can. It was discussed that gut cells and thyroid cells actually originate in the same way. How fascinating is that?

Many "new" studies are being done on the value and purpose of the gut and digestion. I say "new" because it was Hippocrates who said that all illness begins in the gut. Too bad we didn't just listen to him all those centuries ago. Some researchers and physicians are now calling the gut the second brain, but the ones who completely understand the process are calling the gut the actual first brain. For this reason, it is crucial to start to seriously think about the foods we put into our bodies, using supportive digestive enzymes to get the proper nutrients from what we eat, probiotics to keep our gut biome healthy, and supplementation when necessary to give our thyroid extra support to move back into health.

Again, I encourage you to read more at lifeextension.com, but from the thyroid sufferers I have met, as well as caring for the gut, it is crucial to determine if you need a proper form of iodine. To correctly supplement with selenium, zinc, and copper for proper utilization of vitamins, check for iron, B12, and vitamin D deficiencies; check DHEA and pregenolone levels; and explore using herbs such as Guggul extract, L-tyrosine,

Rhodiola, Ashwagandha extract, Korean Ginseng, vitamins A and C.[37] And, in case you have never been warned about the top thyroid disturbers, stay away from chlorine, BPA in plastic, vegetable oils, and if your thyroid is damaged, do become gluten-free, dairy-free, and processed-sugar-free.

The biggest recommendation the thyroid sufferers I interviewed have taught me is that you need both a physician and health coach to look at the whole body, because the doctors who are trained in standard lab work on what a normal thyroid is, diagnosed by potentially faulty lab tests, will keep you from getting the help you desperately need. If nothing else, please read up more on a field called functional medicine and how these physicians are trained to do just that. A good place to start is with Dr. Hyman at http://drhyman.com. These are licensed physicians with a much better feel of how to treat the body—not necessarily with just medications. I hope this information encourages you to learn more. Don't be thrown off by the haters who have tried to say this form of treatment is non-substantiated; keep an open mind and realize that the traditional medical establishment does not have all the information. My best advice to you is to carefully read what these women have suffered through, take whatever information you can from their journey, contact us for more information, and know that we are like-minded with a goal to help you heal from the inside out. As I said in my introduction—I want *you* to lead an exemplary life!

---

[37] "Health Protocols | Life Extension." 2017. *Lifeextension.Com.* http://www.lifeextension. com/Protocols/Metabolic-Health/Thyroid-Regulation/Page-les (accessed January 22, 2017).

Chapter 5

Andrea: Thyroid and Goiter

*The doctor of the future will no longer treat
the human frame with drugs, but rather will
cure and prevent disease with nutrition.*

—*Thomas Edison*

Andrea

It was in one of my Health Coach Training Program lectures at the Institute for Integrative Nutrition that I first met Andrea. I heard her tell her story in two different lectures in fact, and it was so powerful that it stayed with me. Andrea's story pushed me to actually begin planning this book. It gave me so much inspiration and I knew there were many, many other stories out in the world that were just as impactful. People *are* changing their health and thus their lives with nutrition. It's then I knew I could write these stories to give people hope.

Like many young women in our society today, Andrea spent much of her younger years dieting. She tried them all and even referred to herself as a chronic dieter. She ate what she thought was healthy. You know, the low-fat, no-fat stuff that was flooding the markets back in the '90s. It was assumed by most that if something was low in fat then it was good for you. If it didn't have fat in it, then you wouldn't get fat. A huge misconception, even today, is that eating fat makes you fat.

A Senate hearing back in 1976 led to the first set of dietary guidelines for Americans. The critical part of the message got lost in translation though, and what people heard was "stop eating the fat and eat more carbohydrates." What was meant by "carbohydrates" was whole grains, vegetables, and fruits. What ended up happening was the food industry took advantage and created a whole new fad. Americans started eating more highly refined carbs, like fat-free muffins, which were loaded with sugar and processed chemicals to take the place of the removed fat. Well, guess what? When we started eating these highly refined grains and sugars, we as a country started getting fatter. And more diabetic.[38]

There is a lot of controversy about fat and sugar, what's good for us and what is not so good for us, and how much we should or shouldn't have in our daily diets. The truth is that the human body needs fat in order to function properly. We need much less sugar than most people consume. But that could be the topic for a whole other book. Suffice it to say that the human body was not created to live on toxic fabricated, modified, carcinogenic morsels lacking in any nutrition whatsoever.

---

38 "Why We Got Fatter During the Fat-Free Food Boom." 2017. *NPR.Org*. http://www. npr.org/sections/thesalt/2014/03/28/295332576/why-we-got-fatter-during-the-fat-free-food-boom (accessed September 25, 2015).

So Andrea, like many of us, followed what we all believed to be helpful, healthful guidelines. She dieted and lost weight. She did this over and over. All the diets worked, but only for a while; then the weight would creep back up. Nothing stuck for very long.

Andrea would start her day with either boxed cereal and skim or low-fat milk, or a plain bagel with nothing on it. There was always a very large cup of coffee with NutraSweet and soymilk. Lunch was a salad or pizza (without the cheese) and one or two diet Pepsis. A typical dinner back then was a tuna-fish sandwich or soup with some non-fat graham crackers or cookies. Andrea also ate a lot of candy.

All those low-fat, no-fat, and refined foods became the staples of Andrea's diet. Foods in colorful packaging that were highly refined, filled with sugar and chemicals, and not very healthy—some of them even carcinogenic. She had a dieting mindset that unbeknownst to her was destroying her body. Andrea says she was setting herself up for failure—at every single meal. At 28, it happened. She was diagnosed with hyperthyroidism.

Hyperthyroidism is a condition where the thyroid is over-active, produces too much thyroid hormone, and things start going wonky. But, even though she was diagnosed with hy-perthyroid, Andrea was suffering from all of the symptoms of hypothyroid as well. For example, she felt tired and cold frequently, and she had a slow metabolism with a tendency to gain weight. The symptoms are not always the same for every-one with this condition. The one constant that doctors will tell you is that it's incurable.

With both hyperthyroidism and hypothyroidism, a goiter sometimes occurs, which appears as a large mass or lump or swelling in the area of the thyroid. Andrea had a goiter on the front of her neck, and it was visibly obvious to anyone she came across.[39]

Imagine this for a moment. Andrea was 28, a beautiful young woman with a goiter. She even jokingly called herself "Goiter-girl." Imagine how she felt, though, walking around in public. You know how people are—they try not to stare. They look when they think you can't see them. Kids, on the other hand, might outright point and are probably afraid; there is general misunderstanding. I'm cringing just writing this. Imagine the thoughts this young woman had about her appearance; imagine how this impacted her confidence, her sense of worth, her ability to function in today's society. Fortunately, Andrea is stronger than most. She has an internal strength she attributes to her mom that took over and enabled her to do whatever was necessary to heal herself. She said it didn't bother her too much, although she did have one friend who called her "the neck."

Andrea's doctor told her she could not heal this autoimmune disease unless she literally killed her thyroid with radioactive iodine and then took prescription thyroid medication for the rest of her life. She questioned this and asked about nutrition; would it help if she changed her diet? According to her doctor, her thyroid had nothing to do with her diet. Really?

---

39   James Norman, MD, FACE. 2017. "Hypothyroidism: Overview, Causes, and Symptoms." *Endocrineweb*. http://www.endocrineweb.com/conditions/thyroid/hypothyroidism-too-little-thyroid-hormone (accessed September 25, 2015).

In fact, four doctors told her she could not heal this with nutrition. They told her she couldn't heal herself with diet and exercise. She certainly could not heal her body with her mind and self-love.

Well, Andrea seriously didn't like the sound of this. Who would? Radioactive iodine? Seriously? Put that in my body? No way.

Andrea knew instinctively that there was a different way. A better way. A better way for her. She decided to take things into her own hands, went against her doctors' advice, and changed her diet. She chose to not take the radioactive iodine to destroy her thyroid.

Instead, she focused on whole, real food. She questioned everything she had been eating prior to this diagnosis. Andrea knew her entire dietary lifestyle had to change. So, she completely gave up the diet soda and all the prepackaged colorful boxes you find in the center aisles of the supermarket and concentrated on wholesome foods that came directly from the earth.

As an aside, in case you have not yet realized, grocery stores are set up to have the healthy fruits and vegetables, seafood, meats, etc., on outside aisles and junk and processed food on inside aisles. Why? A marketing tool. Most people who run into a store to shop start in the center because they are attracted to the multitude of choices and colorful boxes. Now try to tell me the powers-that-be want us to *be* healthy. People who have caught on to this and want to get healthy "perimeter" shop.

Back to Andrea. A funny thing happened once she stopped eating all the junk food, all the chemicals and the crap sweeteners and focused on whole, real food: she lost eighteen pounds in four months. She wasn't trying to lose the weight—it just came off. She even joked that this thyroid disease was coming in handy! When you change your diet, your body begins to change, but in addition to that—your mind begins to change. You begin to think more clearly. That brain fog disappears. Mental clarity and focus become the norm.

After four months, Andrea went back for blood tests to see how she was doing. The test results indicated that her change in diet was definitely helping and her hormone levels were no longer "dangerously high." However, her doctor said that even though her numbers had improved, they were not within the normal range and she still needed medication. I personally do not understand this. In four months' time she went from dangerously high to just above normal—and her doctor had no reaction except to say that she still needed medication? Really? How about waiting another four months and seeing where the numbers are then?

Well, that's exactly what Andrea did. For two years. She focused on food, on self-care and healing her body. Andrea had patience. She knew that her thyroid condition didn't happen overnight. It took 28 years to manifest in her body; she wasn't going to be cured in a few months. Healing requires patience, which Andrea had in spades.

Over this two-year period, Andrea went back for blood tests every few months, often with a different doctor to get a second and third opinion. Her numbers always improved, but if they weren't in the "normal" range, each doctor would recommend a new prescription medication to manage her symptoms. Never to cure or heal, only to minimize symptoms. She refused every time and continued on her path to healing her body in her own way.

After two years Andrea no longer had a goiter. And her thyroid numbers were normal. She had healed her body with food and with love and with a lot of self-care.

So what did Andrea do exactly? In terms of her diet, she eliminated chemicals, highly refined foods, soda, sugar substitutes, anything artificial, diet foods, fat-free and low-fat foods (if you can call that food), hydrogenated fats such as margarine, white flour, and most dairy products. She focused on organic and clean foods and added vegetables, sea vegetables such as seaweed, whole grains, fish, and small amounts of lean animal proteins. In addition to her dietary changes, Andrea incorporated meditation and daily physical exercise, such as yoga or taking a walk. These particular yoga poses will stimulate the thyroid and bring energy to the throat area: camel pose (*Ustrasana*), bridge pose (*Setu Bandha Sarvangasana*), shoulder stand (*Salamba Sarvangasana*), and plow (*Halasana*).[40]

In contrast to her "before" diet, Andrea now begins her day with things like rice and vegetable porridge or miso salmon soup with shitake mushrooms. Lunch might be a stir-fry with buckwheat noodles or rice, vegetables, and egg; dinner consists of some combination of beans, fish, vegetables, greens, soup, and grains.

---

40 "Speak Your Inner Truth with the Fifth Chakra." 2017. *The Chopra Center*. http://www.chopra.com/articles/speak-your-inner-truth-with-the-fifth-chakra (accessed September 25, 2015).

Something else Andrea did was to focus on her fifth chakra, which is in the thyroid area, and she learned how to use her voice. As she was healing, Andrea shared her journey and her version of the truth, as it relates to healing the body, through writing books and doing lectures. This practice of expressing yourself from a higher form of communication strengthens the fifth chakra. When your fifth chakra is in alignment, you accept your originality, express your authentic voice, and speak your truth. Blocked chakras can lead to illness, so it's important to keep that energy flowing freely.[41]

> "When I had my goiter I was lacking the ability to speak my truth. I used to swallow my words. Now, I healthfully express myself. And, it's made all the difference in the world."

Here are some additional tips for good thyroid health, although these are good tips for everyone who wants to enjoy good health!

Choose organic and clean foods. If you're not eating organic, then you are feeding your body all the pesticides, fungicides, and herbicides that are traditionally used on conventional farms to kill bugs and allow the plants to thrive. Think about this, though: if these things are meant to kill living things, it's only a matter of time before they begin to interfere with our bodily functions. For the thyroid specifically, pesticides, etc., are endocrine disruptors. Simply put, the endocrine system is the body's network of hormone-managing glands, which control bodily functions. The thyroid is one of these glands, which happens to regulate metabolism.[42]

---

41   Ibid.
42   Robert M. Sargis, MD, PhD. 2017. "About the Endocrine System." *Endocrineweb.* http://www.endocrineweb.com/endocrinology/about-endocrine-system (accessed September 25, 2015).

Andrea also recommends eating locally and seasonally. When you eat foods grown locally, you are supporting local farms, boosting the economy, and building more connected communities. This may be obvious, but it also means the foods are traveling less, which translates into less fuel usage and fewer greenhouse gases generated, so it's also good for the environment. The food itself, however, is fresher and has more flavor. Think about this. It doesn't have to spend weeks or months on a ship or tractor-trailer to get from wherever it was grown to you. Typically, foods that have to be shipped from afar (because they are out of season in your local area) are picked before they are ripe, which means they are not given enough time to absorb as many nutrients from the soil. When you eat locally grown foods, they are fresher because they are picked at their peak. Additionally, seasonal foods are in alignment with the environment in which they were grown. According to Andrea, "eating out of season and/or out of climate sends mixed messages to your internal system, throwing the thyroid and endocrine system out of balance."[43,44,45,46]

When it comes to choosing animal proteins, you want to focus on naturally and pasture-raised livestock. These animals are able to roam freely in their natural environment. They are essentially stress-free and live a happy, high-quality life. Factory or conventionally farmed animals, on the other hand, live in deplorable conditions where they have little to

---

43 "10 Reasons Why You Should Eat Local." 2017. *Ecowatch*. http://www.ecowatch.com/10-reasons-why-you-should-eat-local-1882029859.html (accessed September 25, 2015).
44 "Radiate My Thyroid? What?! No Freakin' Way! – Andrea Beaman." 2017. *Andrea Beaman*. http://andreabeaman.com/radiate-my-thyroid-what-no-freakin-way/ (accessed September 25, 2015).
45 "10 Reasons Why You Should Eat Local." 2017. *Ecowatch*. http://www.ecowatch.com/10-reasons-why-you-should-eat-local-1882029859.html (accessed September 25, 2015).
46 Ibid.

no access to the outdoors and sunlight, and many barely have room to breathe. Think about the constant stress in their bodies. Would you want to absorb that kind of energy?[47]

It is scary how true the phrase "you are what you eat" is. If you want to be healthy, support and strengthen your genes, and stay away from doctors, take it from Andrea—it starts from what goes in your mouth.

Advice:

Andrea believes that food is medicine. She will tell you to avoid all "diets," fads, or "isms" and focus on delicious foods that are local, seasonal, and organic. She also believes that nourishment does not only come in the form of food. "When our body, spirit, and emotions work together, we can enjoy vibrant health, boundless energy, and look and feel great."

Inspiration:

Today, Andrea considers herself healthy, and although still in the process of healing, she is confident in her body's ability to heal. She says that when you give your body what it needs, it shows up for you in amazing ways.

My attitude is good. I'm alive and happy and healthy. It's a nice way to live in the world.

---

47   2017. http://www.sustainabletable.org/248/sustainable-livestock-husbandry (accessed September 25, 2015).

Contact:

Andrea is a natural food chef, a certified holistic health counselor, and she hosts a television cooking show called Fed Up! She healed herself with nutrition and self-love and now helps others heal themselves with her coaching practice. She is on a mission to change the health of the planet.

If you want more information about thyroid health or want to get in touch with Andrea, check out her website: http://andreabeaman.com/

Chapter 6

Stephanie: Thyroid and Non-Cancerous Nodules

The food you eat can be the safest form of medicine or the slowest form of poison.

—Anne Wigmore

Stephanie

Sixteen years ago, when Stephanie was pregnant with her daughter she developed high blood pressure, which in her third trimester, developed into preeclampsia. Every parent has heard this term before and it probably sounds scarier than it is, but it is scary nonetheless. Besides hypertension, it comes with higher levels of protein in the urine and swelling, especially in the feet, legs, and hands. As you can imagine, this adds more discomfort to an already uncomfortable body. According to Dr. Weil and other trusted sources, the treatment for preeclampsia is delivery, and Stephanie's daughter had to come a little early.[48,49] Fortunately, everything went well.

After her daughter's birth, however, Stephanie found herself diagnosed with hypothyroidism. The interesting thing, though, was that her doctor didn't bring this to Stephanie's attention. It was her daughters' pediatrician who first noticed that she was gaining a lot of weight. This was the biggest indicator that something was not quite right. Stephanie had regained almost all of her pregnancy weight and in a much shorter amount of time.

While the weight gain was concerning to Stephanie, it was the rate at which she had put it on that was most worrying to her daughter's pediatrician. She advised Stephanie to get herself checked out and get some blood work done. Stephanie's primary care physician, after seeing her blood test results, told Stephanie that she had hypothyroidism and prescribed thyroid medication.

Imagine this for a moment. You just gave birth, which is totally exciting by itself. Then there is the added eagerness of getting your body back. Back from the glorious invasion of another tiny human and back into some semblance of shapeliness. Now imagine that instead of shedding that baby weight—you gain even more. What?

48 Wellness, Health, Mind & Spirit Body, and Pregnancy Fertility. 2017. "Preeclampsia – Dr. Weil." *Drweil.Com.* http://www.drweil.com/health-wellness/body-mind-spirit/pregnancy-fertility/preeclampsia/ (accessed May 6, 2017).
49 Boey, Bernard. 2017. "Maternal-Fetal Medicine | Obstetrics and Gynecology | Weill Cornell Medical College." *Cornellobgyn.Org.* http://www.cornellobgyn.org/clinical_services/maternal_fetal_medicine.html (accessed May 6, 2017).

This was Stephanie. She was gaining weight and she was in a fragile emotional state. Who wouldn't be? This was incomprehensible for her, especially adding the fact that someone else had to point it out. It made her feel that something was seriously wrong. Back then she had never seen or heard of other women having these types of issues post-partum. It wasn't until a few years later when she went back into the corporate world and began having conversations with other women that she realized she wasn't alone. Many women have had similar issues.

When she had her daughter, however, she was alone. Her friends weren't having children when Stephanie was having children. Many of her friends began families a little later in life, whereas Stephanie had them when she was a bit younger. She felt like she was the only person going through this. None of her friends could relate. Apparently, though, gaining weight or continuing to gain weight after giving birth is not uncommon. A Japanese study found that 5 to 10 percent of women who are pregnant develop issues with inflammation in the thyroid, which can lead to weight gain after giving birth. Lack of sleep and stress, both of which many new moms experience, also contribute to weight gain. Stephanie was definitely not alone.[50]

After six months, her doctor slowly weaned her off the thyroid medication and she was fine for a little while, but then Stephanie noticed she was gaining weight again. It was at this point that Stephanie came across the book *Skinny Bitch* by

---

50 2017. http://www.modernmom.com/2c3cf2b0-051f-11e2-9d62-404062497d7e.htm (accessed November 25, 2015).

Rory Freedman and Kim Barnouin. The book guides women to a healthy, clean-eating lifestyle in a laugh-out-loud, no-holds-barred kind of way. This was the first thing that Stephanie ever read that got into the heart of what has happened to our food in this country. It covers things like what's in our food, how animals are treated in conventional farming methods, the difference between proteins and carbohydrates, the dangers of soda and sugar, and the importance of pooping, among other things. Stephanie described the book as an in-your-face exposition on why people have health problems.

It made so much sense to her, and Stephanie was sick and tired of feeling sick and tired. This particular book opened her eyes to all the different things that are wrong with our food and she got very angry. This fueled her motivation to change. She decided then and there that she would do whatever she could to release the excess weight and stop eating all the garbage. Stephanie went "cold turkey" and gave up all animal proteins. She became not quite vegan, but was full vegetarian and continued to eat small quantities of cheese and eggs. Along with her change in diet, Stephanie started working out because she was tired of feeling terrible all the time.

But, Stephanie went a little overboard and attacked her weight a bit too aggressively. She was exercising a lot and eating too little—to the point where she lost 75 pounds in about two months. That is extreme! Seriously extreme! Stephanie realized she was doing something right and at the same time doing something not so right. At her lowest weight, Stephanie was 98 pounds. This was unacceptable to her and she understood that it was not healthy. This rapid weight loss put a huge stress on her body and she developed anemia, which is a lack of red blood cells. When your body has too few red blood cells, it doesn't get enough oxygen and organs stop functioning properly. If left unattended, this can lead to serious complications.[51]

During this time, Stephanie also had a non-cancerous nodule that formed on her thyroid. Most of the time, these types of nodules don't cause problems and don't even require treatment. Her doctor was a bit concerned, however, because sometimes if they continue to grow, they can cause problems with breathing. Stephanie was lucky and had no issues with her nodule, and while she still has it today, it has decreased in size and it is completely unnoticeable.

According to Stephanie, the nodule formed on the side of her thyroid that had stopped working, and when the nodule took up shop, it began to act as a mini-thyroid and balanced everything out. Her ear, nose, and throat (ENT) specialist and her endocrinologist had both suggested having this nodule removed. Stephanie refused. She felt there was no reason to take it out if her thyroid levels were normal.

As a unique bio-individual human, Stephanie was performing all sorts of experiments with her diet and body, which is a good thing. Who is going to understand your body and its needs better than anyone else? You! We are all unique human beings and we all have unique dietary requirements. Stephanie called herself her own guinea pig when it comes to health. Going through this experience led her to know that

---

51   Wellness, Health, and Mind & Spirit Body. 2017. "Anemia – Dr. Weil's Condition Care Guide." *Drweil.Com*. http://www.drweil.com/health-wellness/body-mind-spirit/heart/anemia (accessed February 5, 2017).

her body needs animal proteins. She learned that the various vegan protein options don't give her body what it needs and that animal proteins make her feel better.

So, she went back to eating meat and continued to exclude junk food and dairy. She also started reading about thyroid health, healing the gut, and the body's endocrine system, which are all connected. She first paid attention to healing her gut and started juicing, taking probiotics, and eating gutheal-ing foods with natural probiotics in them—things like real yo-gurt, on occasion, and naturally fermented sauerkraut. She also added foods with fiber. Stephanie focused on lots of fruits and vegetables, all organic and free of pesticides, to help her body detox and promote lymph flow.[52]

Along with her change in diet, Stephanie concentrated on other ways of reducing stress in her life.[53] For example, in the past she was a runner, did lots of cardio and very fast-moving types of sports. Now she took up yoga, which is a great way to reduce stress, increase balance and flexibility, and lower blood pressure as well as cortisol levels. Yoga and juicing was the combination that helped Stephanie turn her health around for the longer term.

That was sixteen years ago. Sixteen years of being on track to healing her thyroid and endocrine system. It's been a long journey and has definitely not been easy, but Stephanie found

52 "Clean Your Body's Drains: 10 Ways to Detoxify Your Lymphatic System." 2017. *Healthy and Natural World.* http://www.healthyandnaturalworld.com/natural-ways-to-cleanse-your-lymphatic-system/ (accessed November 25, 2015).

53 Wellness, Health, Mind & Spirit Body, and Stress Anxiety. 2017. "Reduce Stress – Dr. Weil." *Drweil.Com.* http://www.drweil.com/health-wellness/body-mind-spirit/stress-anxiety/ten-ways-to-reduce-stress (accessed February 5, 2017).

what works for her body. Today, she does not take any thyroid medications. None. She gets her blood tested every year and her thyroid is steady. Her numbers remain well within normal range.

Stephanie still continues to live healthfully with her change in diet and lifestyle. She is so happy that she doesn't have to take any thyroid medications. Healing her thyroid was critical. When you don't have a thyroid making those hormones for you, you require thyroid medication. You cannot survive without it. This is very scary to Stephanie—to have to rely on a medication to live. Not to mention possible side effects of taking thyroid medications, which include sleep problems, hair loss, muscle or joint pain, swelling, itching, minor skin rashes, nausea, stomach cramps, diarrhea, and constipation. Thyroid medications can also interact with other drugs you might be taking and can interact negatively with calcium, fiber, and walnuts. Something else to think about is that the ingredients in thyroid medication—and pretty much any medication—include things like cornstarch, lactose, and artificial coloring.[54] Getting healthy is about getting rid of artificial toxins, so why would we want these ingredients in our medication?

Thankfully, Stephanie was able to heal her thyroid and avoid a lifetime of thyroid medication, much like Andrea Beaman in the chapter before. Stephanie considers Andrea an inspiration. She confirmed and validated for Stephanie everything she is doing for her thyroid and overall health.

---

54 "What Are the Common Side Effects and Interactions of Thyroid Medication?" 2017. *Naturalendocrinesolutions.Com*. http://www.naturalendocrinesolutions.com/articles/common-side-effects-interactions-thyroid-medication/ (accessed November 25, 2015).

Back when Stephanie was pregnant with her daughter, her diet was not the best. She described it as that typical pregnant woman who thought she could eat whatever she wanted. For example, she would eat ice cream. A lot of ice cream! Subway sandwiches and chips were her favorite meal; she would eat those almost every day. And, her family ate a lot of fast food. At the time, Stephanie and her husband owned their own business and were constantly busy. Especially after her daughter was born. Fast food was quick, easy, and convenient. While she understood it wasn't healthy, it filled a need.

Today, Stephanie's diet is much healthier. She tries to eat as many whole foods as she can. She describes it this way: "If you can't grow it or get it out in nature, we don't eat it." Water and clean eating have become a way of life. Stephanie's diet is also gluten free. She used to have stomach issues, which is what led her to research about healing her gut. When she used to eat, she would feel horrible and sometimes double over in pain. Stephanie recalled that these stomach issues dated back to when she was a child. She always remembers having pain. It's not something she recognized way back then, but as she reduced gluten and began feeling better, the memories of childhood came back. Now that she is totally gluten free, she has none of those symptoms anymore.

Breakfast cycles between smoothies and juices. Stephanie noted that when she juiced every day she didn't feel the same effect, so she alternates with juicing one day and a smoothie the next. She describes herself as an all-or-nothing kind of person, and when she first started juicing, she did it religiously every single day. For a long time it made her feel great; she had that amazing nutrient boost that she would feel almost immediately. However, after doing this for a year every single day, she wasn't feeling that same effect.

Her every-other-day breakfast smoothies consist of frozen banana and almond milk (the kind without carrageenan) as the base, and then depending on how she's feeling she'll add a variety of cacao, peanut butter, dates (for sweetness and iron), fruit, maca, hemp seeds, matcha tea, etc. Lunch typically includes a salad with a bunch of vegetables or a gluten-free wrap with black beans, sprouts, avocado, and greens with a vegan chipotle mayonnaise made from avocados.

As a side note, carrageenan is a natural common food additive that is extracted from a red seaweed, Chondrus crispus, popularly known as Irish moss. Carrageenan, which has no nutritional value, has been used as a thickener and emulsifier to improve the texture of ice cream, yogurt, cottage cheese, soymilk, and other processed foods. It can cause problems with some people, as the human body doesn't know how to process it, which can lead to inflammation. Studies have been linking carrageenan to health issues, such as ulcerative colitis, gastrointestinal ulcers, and colon cancer for over fifty years.[55]

Some animal studies have linked degraded forms of carrageenan (the type not used in food) to ulcerations and cancers of the gastrointestinal tract. More worrisome, undegraded carrageenan—the type that is widely used in foods—has been associated with malignancies and other stomach problems.

---

[55] 2017. *Isitbadforyou.Com.* https://www.isitbadforyou.com/questions/is-carrageenan-bad-for-you (accessed November 25, 2015).

In 2012, Joanne K. Tobacman, MD, who has published multiple peer-reviewed studies about the biological effects of carrageenan, addressed the National Organic Standards Board on this issue and urged reconsideration of the use of carrageenan in organic foods. According to Dr. Tobacman, her research has shown that exposure to carrageenan causes inflammation, and that when we consume processed foods containing it, we ingest enough to cause inflammation in our bodies. That's a problem since chronic inflammation is a root cause of many serious diseases including heart disease, Alzheimer's and Parkinson's diseases, and cancer.[56] This issue needs more research, but the great news is that with new labeling laws the almond or coconut milk you buy in the store will often say "carrageenan free."

Stephanie tries not to eat meat during the day and then for dinner she'll have salmon, chicken, or beef. Any animal protein she puts into her body is organic and as clean as possible. This is especially important for thyroid health, as conventionally farmed animals may consume feed that contains pesticides, which are endocrine disruptors. This means they can impact the production, release, and metabolism of hormones and stop your thyroid from functioning properly. Stephanie loves potatoes and often mixes sweet and regular potatoes, mashed as a side dish. Dinner always includes some vegetables depending on the season. For example, in autumn, Stephanie roasts root vegetables such as butternut squash with some coconut or almond milk and seasoning.

---

56 Nutrition, Diet, Food Safety, and Q A. 2017. "Carrageenan Dangers – Carrageenan Safety | Dr. Weil." *Drweil.Com.* http://www.drweil.com/diet-nutrition/food-safety/is-carrageenan-safe/ (accessed February 3, 2017).

Other benefits of her change in diet include better skin. Stephanie's skin now has a dewiness that it never had before. Changing her diet changed her life. Literally. She is happy and energetic and enjoys life again. She knows that she has control over her health.

Inspiration:

Stephanie's journey to health taught her so much about how intelligent and miraculous the human body truly is. Your body is amazing! Your body is meant to heal itself. You just have to give it what it needs, whether that's nutrition, sunshine, less stress, or all of the above. Your body speaks to you through pain and other symptoms, but you need to listen! It is because of this that Stephanie is able to regulate her thyroid condition without medication.

Advice:

Stephanie wants you to know that there is always hope. Always. Her closing words were these:

> "I've heard so many stories of and met people who have pulled through debilitating diseases through a commitment to a healthier lifestyle. The statistics are astonishing, and there is no denying them. If you have the willingness to overcome something, you will. I can say that, because I've witnessed this firsthand with my own health issues. Support from family and friends is

also key in sustaining lifestyle changes for the good of your health. Surround yourself with supportive people—those who are willing to go to that yoga class with you or who will try that new gluten-free item on the menu. Lastly, be your own health advocate! You know your body better than anyone else, so ask questions and seek answers that feel right for you."

Contact Info:

Stephanie is a graduate from the Institute of Integrative Nutrition, which equipped her with extensive, cutting-edge knowledge in holistic nutrition, health coaching, and prevention. With this and through her own healing journey, Stephanie developed a passion for helping other women with similar health problems achieve their optimum health. Her approach to wellness is to identify the root cause of health issues and teach you how all areas of your life are connected.

If you want more information about Stephanie, want to work with her, or get in touch with her, check out her website: swell.liveeditaurora.com

PART THREE

Invisible Illness:
Just Because
You Don't See
It Doesn't Mean
It's Not There

Chapter 7

Fibromyalgia, Migraines, Mold and Chemical Sensitives: The Evolution of Our Obsession with Scented Inventions

The longer I live the more I seem to come upon these "unknown" or hidden illnesses that are not visible to the outside world but leave a person suffering nonetheless. They are the ones for which doctors prescribe antidepressants that often have nothing to do with the hidden physical illness the person is suffering from. They are the ones doctors have accusatorily thrown the phrase out to women that "if I don't find something in this next set of tests, I'm going to say it is all in your head." These women are met with disbelief, they are treated poorly, they are not taken seriously, and on top of all the suffering they are already experiencing, this packs a punch so debilitating that it is amazing that anyone can get up and function after dealing with such hurtful and hopeless words.

It is terrible to say, but if you tell people you are diagnosed with a disease that is commonly seen in the media such as high cholesterol, high blood pressure, cancer, diabetes ... you get sympathy and people seem to respond. When you say you are diagnosed with fibromyalgia, Epstein-Barr Virus (EBV), or a biotoxin illness—something people can't see—they think it's all in your mind, or you're just not a strong individual and you're blowing things way out of proportion.

Women have lost their jobs, their families, their relationships, their self-esteem, and so much more from these invisible illnesses. We need to find it in our hearts to not just automatically label them as hypochondriacs and/or weak and realize that more and more of these "undefined" unknown illnesses are popping up because of the toxic environment we live in today.

For years there was an illness known as fibromyalgia, and doctors were not able to pinpoint or even understand that it existed. It was where mostly women (the statistics now say about 9 out of 10) complained of deep, debilitating pain in different sections of their body, but when blood tests came back the person looked perfectly healthy. Some patients were referred to rheumatologists, thinking it might be the start of arthritis or something else, and again, even the specialists would say "you are healthy, it must be in your head." By 1972, however, progress was starting to be made when "Dr. Hugh Smythe laid the foundation for the modern definition of fibromyalgia by describing widespread pain and tender points." Technically, this illness has been around for centuries, but this is when current physicians and teaching hospitals seemed to start to really pay attention to the fact that this might be a real disease![57] "For a disease with no known cause, fibromyalgia sure affects a lot of people, at least 5 million in the U.S. alone. That's about an estimated 2–4% of the population!"[58] Imagine this many people suffering on a daily basis from just one disease.

With fibromyalgia not only does the person feel exhausted, but they have points on their body that are so painful you barely touch the person and they feel like they could jump out of their skin in pain. It is so bad that if, for example, the arm is affected, you can barely pick up a cup or even light clothes without feeling a deep sensation of agony. The thought of living like that is devastating, and I share the story of a woman with newborn twins, Nicole, who could barely hold her daughters to breastfeed because of the pain. For a formal diagnosis of fibromyalgia, you must have pain in 11 out of the 18 tender areas or points. If 11 of 18 tender points are affected, how could anyone function?

As for whether this is genetics or epigenetics, "Increasing evidence supports a strong genetic component to fibromyalgia. Siblings, parents, and children of a person with fibromyalgia are eight times more likely to have fibromyalgia than those who have no relatives with the condition. There are several genes that have been suspected to play a role in fibromyalgia."[59]

57   "History of Fibromyalgia." 2017. *Healthcentral.Com.* http://www.healthcentral.com/chronic-pain/fibromyalgia-287647-5.html (accessed May 6, 2017).
58   2017. "5 Natural Remedies for Fibromyalgia – Draxe.Com." 2017. Dr. Axe. https://draxe.com/natural-remedies-for- fibromyalgia (accessed May 6, 2017).
59   Catherine Burt Driver, MD. 2017. "Fibromyalgia Symptoms, Treatment, Causes – Is Fibromyalgia Hereditary? – Medicinenet." *Medicinenet.* http://www.medicinenet.com/fibromyalgia_facts/page2.htm (accessed May 6, 2017).

There is some new and mounting evidence that some of these cases are misdiagnosed and are really thyroid issues gone awry or even chemical sensitives and immune-suppressed disorders that can't otherwise be diagnosed. The thing I don't like about these hidden and misdiagnosed illnesses is that they are too easily missed and patients are put on antidepressants, anti-anxiety, sleep medicines, or even antibiotics because the doctor just can't figure out what else to do. Regardless of the illness, the patient is really suffering and has very little quality of life.

The truth is that with all the toxins and chemicals out there, an already toxic body will show itself by giving you, the owner, pain. Think about what happens to your healthy cells when they are constantly bombarded by things like paint fumes, gas fumes, or even mold as you read about Tara and her biotoxin illness. Think about walking down the aisle at a grocery store in the detergent section. How many different smells, or rather scents, come from that aisle? If you have any type of auto-immune disorder, even mononucleosis or Epstein-Barr, then you are going to be affected by these "scents." Think about the crazy car deodorizers people use, the off-gassing from new carpeting, that new leather smell in a new car, the deodorizers that smell like fresh air—yes, you read that correctly. Fresh air, really? You get my point. These chemicals are quietly but effectively weakening our immune systems, and we are worried about nerve toxins being sent from a foreign country? What are we doing to ourselves in our own country? These scents trigger all sorts of illnesses we can't see, but they are deadly nonetheless and can cause anything from fibromyalgia to chemical sensitivities to migraines.

Migraines are actually another example of a completely debilitating illness that can't be seen, but the person affected, I assure you, can't function. Whether it is the raging pressure in the head, the extreme sensitivity to light, the nausea, the vertigo, the inability to function; all these symptoms, quite frankly even just one, knock you out—completely. You will read about Denise, who struggled with them since the age of five. Imagine, five years old. In her case she was predisposed because it turns out her mother and her grandmother suffered from them as well. According to the research, "Single gene disorders that result in migraines are rare. One of these is known as familial hemiplegic migraine, a type of migraine with aura, which is inherited in an autosomal dominant fashion. Four genes have been shown to be involved in familial hemiplegic migraine."[60] Consider her rare, and when you read about her pain you will wonder how she managed to overcome. When you read about any of these women you will be amazed they made it through, and even more they want to help others!

So, read along with compassion for what these women have endured, and if you are going through something similar, this book is created to help you. Reach out to any or all of us for guidance and support, a listening ear, and any help we can provide so that not only are you heard, but you can start to change your life and move towards health. These women offer us all hope and have made it their life's purpose to help you heal; please take them up on their offers and learn from their valuable and encouraging words.

---

60 "Genetics of Migraine Headaches." 2017. *En.Wikipedia.Org*. https://en.wikipedia.org/wiki/Genetics_of_migraine_headaches (accessed February 3, 2017).

Chapter 8

Nicole: Migraines and Fibromyalgia

*The natural healing force within each of us
is the greatest force in getting well. Our food
should be our medicine. Our medicine should
be our food.*

—Hippocrates

Nicole

About fifteen years ago Nicole was hospitalized with symptoms of a stomach bug; she was throwing up, had diarrhea, and her heart rate was elevated. When they did blood work, they told her she had Graves' disease. This is a form of hyperthyroid disease, and in this case it was caused by a virus attacking her thyroid, which caused it to go out of whack.

Often the trigger for hyperthyroidism, Graves' disease causes the thyroid gland to produce more thyroid hormone than the body needs. It's also an autoimmune problem. As we've seen before, this is when your immune system attacks healthy areas of your body and causes disease.[61]

Over a period of years, Nicole started getting symptoms of fibromyalgia, though it took a very long time to diagnose. Fibromyalgia symptoms vary from person to person, typically accumulate over time, and they ebb and flow in cycles. Since the symptoms are so varied, doctors have a difficult time diagnosing it. Nicole feels her thyroid issues triggered this. She started feeling achy all the time, run down, and had periodic bouts of depression. She knew something was wrong, she just didn't know what.

Through the years she kept going back to doctors and rheumatologists, hoping they would figure out what was wrong with her. They would do various tests and some would say she had symptoms of fibromyalgia, but there was nothing specific they could pinpoint. So Nicole kept plugging along.

It is important to interject here that often because of a missed thyroid disorder as discussed in the first part of this book, doctors lump the illnesses that have similar symptoms and label the illness fibromyalgia. When this is your diagnosis, I recommend you keep researching, searching and seeking answers, because there is a very good chance there is something autoimmune going on at a deeper level and you don't want to just treat the symptoms, you want to heal from the core issue. The good news is that Nicole kept looking.

61   Daniel J. Toft, MD, PhD. 2017. "Graves' Disease Overview." *Endocrineweb*. https://www.endocrineweb.com/conditions/graves-disease/graves-disease-overview (accessed January 31, 2017).

Nicole had her girls (twins, now seven years old) through in vitro fertilization. Nicole believes it was the in vitro that really brought on the fibromyalgia—specifically the chemicals being put into her body and the strain of carrying twins. After having them it flared up, and that was the worst time she ever had.

She was at a point where the doctors wanted to put her on medication, and since she now had twin baby girls, Nicole didn't feel comfortable taking any prescribed medications, especially the antidepressants they wanted her to take. She was so afraid that she would have an adverse reaction to taking antidepressants and wouldn't be able to function. I think we'd all agree—with a newborn it's of key importance to be as healthy as possible. Imagine having newborn *twins* and not being able to function!

It was extremely difficult for Nicole. She was in a lot of pain. She was run down. Her body ached. You could hardly touch her. Her experience was mostly in her upper body, so it was difficult for her to be touched on her arms or hands, etc. Imagine trying to hold newborn infants when your arms and hands are constantly hurting!

In order to be diagnosed with fibromyalgia today, according to Andrew Weil, MD, patients have to have "pain in four quadrants of the body for a minimum of three months and tenderness in at least 11 of 18 specific areas called "tender points" on the neck, shoulders, back, hips, arms or legs that hurt when touched."[62] Nicole certainly had that!

---

62 Wellness, Health, Mind & Spirit Body, and Autoimmune Disorders. 2017. "What Is Fibromyalgia? Fibromyalgia Treatment – Dr. Weil." *Drweil.Com.* http://www.drweil.com/health-wellness/body-mind-spirit/autoimmune-disorders/fibromyalgia/ (accessed February 3, 2017).

It was horrible. There were days when she had to call her husband in the middle of the day to come home from work because she couldn't bear the pain. Physically, Nicole was always achy. She felt like she had the flu all the time. She would get up and do a few things, and then she would have to sit back down and rest for a while before moving on to the next thing. Carrying the laundry was sometimes too much for her. Her joints would be screaming. Nicole described it like this: "Underneath the skin was on fire. So if anyone touches you, even in the slightest way, it hurts." That was the physical aspect of it.

Fibromyalgia also affects the brain, so Nicole was often in a fog. There were times when she would be doing something and in an instant totally forget what she was going to do next. Brain fog was a way of life. On top of that, your hormones and your body in general are thrown off, so depression may sink in. There were times Nicole just wanted to sleep, times when she didn't want to deal with life. It's a combination of physical and mental debilitation, and Nicole said the more you give in to it, the more it sucks you down.

When you have fibromyalgia and you don't know any better, it's just a way of life. You learn to cope and it creates a new norm. When you have any illness for a long period, it becomes difficult to change the way you think. You surrender to it; you wake up every day and wonder, *Okay, what's today going to bring me?* Throw in twins on top of that and you get a picture of Nicole's life. It was a challenge. Every. Single. Day. She obviously had to take care of her girls, even when she had debilitating pain. She also had to push herself.

Nicole reflected that besides the chemicals from three rounds of in vitro fertilization, she worked in the hair industry for 25 years. That's 25 years surrounded by toxic fumes. All day long. Add to that carrying twins for nine months, and I think we can all assume her hormones were off the wall.

Her body was out of whack, as she put it, with all the chemicals and toxins coursing through her system. Back then she had very little understanding of what this even meant. How many people understand how toxic they are and how the body reacts to being toxic?

Most of us go through life thinking as long as we eat healthy and organic and avoid fast food, we're okay. This is far from the truth. Think about it. There are pollutants in our air; there are pollutants in our water; we use toxic chemicals to clean our homes; there are toxic fumes emanating from our couches and carpeting and flooring and even our mattresses. Women wear makeup and dye their hair—all toxic! Even deodorant and toothpaste can be harmful to our bodies. We are constantly bombarded with toxins and impurities, to the point that our body's natural filters often become so clogged they can't keep up. Our bodies need help getting those impurities out of our systems.

Fibromyalgia also impacts mood, and Nicole frequently had mood swings on top of everything else. Thankfully a friend of hers introduced her to a nutritional cleansing program. Her friend explained what it was all about, including the nutrition and proper absorption aspect. Nicole, always cautious, went to talk to her doctor about it. He had heard of it as a weight loss system and wasn't sure it was going to help Nicole's fibromyalgia symptoms. Nicole knew she had to try something, though, because taking medication was not an option for her.

She started with a 30-day system, and within about a week or so, her inflammation started decreasing and she started feeling more alive. And not so much like she was dragging a weight on her back all the time.

After the 30 days, Nicole felt like a normal person. *Like a healthy normal person.* Her inflammation had decreased and her aches were minimal. She still does get flare-ups periodically, which she realizes are food related. Like any good patient, Nicole did her research and learned a lot about food as it relates to her particular issues. For example, when you have inflammation, you have to avoid gluten and be very careful with products that have a lot of sodium, etc. She became very aware of things she was putting into her body, what she needed to avoid, and what foods are good to help minimize inflammation.

Low-level or chronic inflammation can lead to more serious conditions, such as heart disease, cancer, and even psychological disorders like depression. According to Dr. Weil, "The extent of this chronic inflammation is influenced by genetics, a sedentary lifestyle, too much stress, and exposure to environmental toxins such as secondhand tobacco smoke. Diet has a huge impact." There are foods, however, that help decrease inflammation, including: organic red wine, a high-quality multivitamin/multimineral, tea, herbs and spices (e.g., turmeric, cinnamon, ginger, garlic, and basil), cooked

Asian mushrooms, fish, shellfish, healthy fats (e.g., olive oil, avocados, walnuts, flaxseed), whole and cracked grains (e.g., brown rice, quinoa, steel-cut oats), beans and legumes, vegetables, fruits, and lots of water throughout the day to flush out toxins.[63]

Adding foods like this to her diet helped Nicole minimize inflammation in her body. Other causes of inflammation include environmental factors, such as pollution, chemicals and airborne irritants, and pesticides. This right here is why it is so important to eat the highest-quality organic food you can afford. Eliminate pesticides and herbicides from your diet at all costs. Inflammation is also a result of stress, physical trauma, and family history. Other things that help reduce inflammation are exercise and specifically yoga and meditation, which promote mental clarity and reduce stress.

Two and a half years later, Nicole is still using the nutritional cleansing products. She loves them and loves how they make her feel. Most of the time. She sometimes gets food, hormone, and/or weather-related flare-ups, but overall her inflammation has definitely decreased and she's able to function on an everyday basis. Like a "normal" person.

These products have helped her tremendously. They were designed to help support our systems' natural functions. Made with the purest-quality undenatured whey protein, active enzymes, botanicals, vitamins, minerals, plant-based adaptogens, and natural cleansing herbs, they help boost metabolism

---

63   Nutrition, Diet, Anti-Inflammatory Pyramid, and Dr. Pyramid. 2017. "Dr. Weil's Anti-Inflammatory Food Pyramid | Anti-Inflammatory Foods." *Drweil.Com.* http://www.drweil.com/diet-nutrition/anti-inflammatory-diet-pyramid/dr-weils-anti-inflammatory-food-pyramid (accessed February 3, 2017).

and energy, protect cells from aging, boost mental clarity, and support detoxification. Whether we realize it or not with the toxic world we live in—everyone needs this!

Her transformation has become her passion. Nicole is on a mission to help other women and moms understand that we don't have to feel sick and tired all the time because our bodies are designed to feel amazing. That we are not supposed to be tired at 3 pm, or wake up tired after not sleeping well. It's been a blessing. Nicole found something natural to help with her symptoms and was able to avoid prescription medication. She is so very happy to be able to control the inflammation and can't imagine what she would be like if she hadn't found nutritional cleansing.

The changes Nicole experienced as a result of using these products run the gamut. They have helped her change tremendously in terms of health, but also mentally, physically, and even spiritually. When you find something like these nutritional cleansing products and you're in a community of positive, like-minded people, you have to change the way you think. It helps you push yourself.

Her diet used to consist of anything she wanted. Nicole was a big carb junkie and would eat pasta constantly. Can you say gluten? Since she worked in the beauty industry, she was on the run all the time, so lunch was whatever she could throw down the fastest, like sandwiches. Chicken parmesan sandwiches in particular. It was definitely not a healthy lifestyle.

Today Nicole's diet is mostly free of gluten. She says it's not 100% as it's often difficult to avoid, but she very carefully watches her gluten intake. When she does ingest gluten, she adds more of the nutritional cleansing products to her day to help with the inflammation. In general, she focuses on fresh fruits, fresh vegetables, lots of water—this is crucial for someone with inflammation! It's so good to flush out whatever we've built up during the day. She also eats a lot of salads, grilled organic chicken, and all-natural foods, meaning not processed.

As no one is perfect, Nicole does "cheat" sometimes, but she pays for it the next day. It's a constant reminder for her to eat well and listen to her body.

One of her girls loves the meal-replacement shakes and often has it for breakfast. Her other daughter loves the bars, which are made with the same nutrient makeup for the most part. This is a bonus of this program—everyone in the family can use the products. Both the bars and the meal-replacement shakes are chock-full of amazing nutrients to fuel your day.

Nicole's mom, Marcia, has rheumatoid arthritis (another autoimmune disease), polymyalgia (another inflammation-related illness causing muscle pain and stiffness in areas typically in the hips and upper body), and spinal stenosis (a narrowing of open spaces in the spine which may cause pain, tingling, and/or numbness).[64,65] She was in worse shape than Nicole was. For over a year now, though, she has been using

64 Wellness, Health, Health Centers, Aging Gracefully, and Q A. 2017. "Treating Polymyalgia Rheumatica? – Drweil.Com." *Drweil.Com*. http://www.drweil.com/health-wellness/health-centers/aging-gracefully/treating-polymyalgia-rheumatica/ (accessed February 3, 2017).

65 "Spinal Stenosis – Mayo Clinic." 2017. *Mayo Clinic*. http://www.mayoclinic.org/diseases-conditions/spinal-stenosis/basics/definition/CON-20036105 (accessed February 3, 2017).

the same nutritional cleansing products and has seen huge improvements in her inflammation and her C-reactive protein (CRP) level. An elevated CRP level indicates increased inflammation in the body. Marcia's CRP number has come down so much so that her doctor took her off steroids. She doesn't even take any rheumatoid arthritis (RA) medication anymore. [66] She follows a healthier diet, uses the nutritional cleansing products, and once in a while takes some pain medication. How awesome is that!

Recent research is finding that autoimmune diseases can be genetically related. According to Ramos, Shedlock, and Langefeld, "It is the general consensus that there is a common genetic background predisposing to autoimmunity."[67] Thus it's not surprising to hear about Nicole's mom. Nicole feels there is definitely a link seeing that both she and her mom have related issues.

Inspiration:

For Nicole, this journey was worth the pain. She has found her tribe of like-minded people. The community of men and women in the nutritional cleansing world and specifically on her team inspire her. They helped her change the way she thinks, and this enabled Nicole to find her true inner self. She

---

66   Wellness, Health, and Mind & Spirit Body. 2017. "Elevated C-Reactive Protein – CRP – Symptoms, Causes & Treatments." *Drweil.Com.* http://www.drweil.com/health-wellness/body-mind-spirit/heart/elevated-c-reactive-protein-crp (accessed February 3, 2017).

67   2017. http://www.nature.com/jhg/journal/v60/n11/full/jhg201594a.html (accessed March 3, 2017).

has figured out who she wants to be and has a much more positive attitude. As much as your body hurts, you still have to go through each day. You can't allow the fibromyalgia to take over—you have to take control of it. Whatever it is you are fighting, you can't let it take control.

She still has rough days. The day of our interview was one such day. She was PMSing, so her hormones were off, which flares her fibromyalgia. Plus it was a much colder day, which is difficult for her. Days like this would make the "old" Nicole want to climb back into bed. Or curl up on the couch with a warm blanket. Not the new Nicole. No, she was still going to her Tae Kwon Do class. She pushes herself, especially on the more difficult days. Nicole knows she will feel better if she gets her body moving. That's what she holds onto.

Advice:

Her advice? Don't allow your physical pain and mental pain to be your jail, your prison. Allow it to be your platform to push forward and conquer what you need to conquer. Just know there is a brighter side. Having to find the one person or message or solution to help you change your mental state is the key. When you are in the darkest of times and you don't want to hear people or you think there is nothing that's going to make a difference, you have to connect with your higher power. Connect with your higher self, in whatever way resonates with you. Whether it's through spirituality, a television show, meditation, yoga, a book, or a person, find that something. Nicole has definitely become more spiritual and has opened herself to more positive things in her life.

Contact:

If you've been inspired by Nicole's story, want to contact her, or want more information on her nutritional cleansing program, you can call her at 973-202-2920, or send her an email at nikkie06210@gmail.com

Chapter 9

Tara: Biotoxin Illness and the Hidden Dangers of Mold

We need role models who are going to break the mold.

—Carly Simon

Tara

Growing up, Tara lived the typical American lower-income family lifestyle. There wasn't a lot of money to offer many options, so what she and her family ate was the Standard American Diet (SAD). As we've seen before, this meant a lot of meats, bad fats, and processed foods, and not enough fiber and plant-based foods. Most people don't realize this is not an optimal diet and don't think twice about it.[68]

---

68 Sears, Dr. 2017. "Standard American Diet (SAD) | Ask Dr. Sears." *Ask Dr. Sears | The Trusted Resource for Parents.* http://www.askdrsears.com/topics/feeding-eating/family-nutrition/standard-american-diet-sad (accessed February 9, 2017).

In all other respects, Tara's childhood was good and she has fond memories. Moving into adulthood is when things started to shift for her. She thought she was eating right, based on the way she was raised, though she did begin to explore eating more vegetables and a little less meat. As she moved into her twenties and even her thirties, Tara started to become more serious about her diet—a trend that continues to this day.

She was very healthy, especially between the ages of thirty to thirty-seven. A lover of the outdoors, Tara was frequently exercising out in fresh air. She did all sorts of things like hiking, skiing, biking, and running. She described it as: "Those lovely outdoor activities that give you all kinds of energy and life in your body." Being one with nature is important to Tara.

During this time, Tara thought she was eating really well. She had reduced red meat and pork; she was eating lean; she avoided those no-fat and low-fat things. It was at this point in our conversation that Tara said she thought she was healthy because she hadn't yet *collapsed*. Yeah ... I can't wait for the rest of this story either.

Jumping ahead a couple of years, Tara had a few instances of less than optimal health—for example, kidney stones. Picture this. You're driving on a highway in the fast lane, and all of a sudden you're doubled over in pain with the worst cramps you've ever had in your entire life. You can't pull the car over to the left, as it's extremely dangerous with cars flying by at 80 MPH. Fortunately, Tara was able to move over to the right and saw a hospital sign, which she followed.

She doesn't remember getting to the emergency room. She only remembers seeing the sign for the hospital and knowing the exit was there. She remembers nothing after that until someone found her on the ground of the hospital parking lot. Tara was very toxic and ended up being in the hospital for a week and a half on a heavy dose of antibiotics. Apparently there were a bunch of other things going on besides the kidney stones.

Tara described this as the beginning of her demise, that moment in time after which everything went haywire. The round of antibiotics she was on threw her immune system for a loop. Tara was already sick inside and didn't even know it, until about a year and a half later, in June 2011, when her body just collapsed. She couldn't see and she described the feeling as having the worst vertigo you can imagine, with pain all over.

That lasted a solid six months where she could barely function. Tara went to doctor after doctor. They thought she had Lyme disease and put her on more antibiotics, which did nothing. Unfortunately, this was a false-positive. She did not have Lyme disease, which meant she could stop taking those antibiotics. But, as we all know, antibiotics mess up your gut, so now Tara was dealing with that as well as a severe undiagnosed illness.

The doctor visits continued as they tried more tests to figure it out. They would ask about symptoms and then say, "well it sounds like you have mononucleosis." Then it was the flu. It obviously wasn't the flu as the flu doesn't last for three months! Tara couldn't go to work, she couldn't drive a car, and she couldn't walk without assistance. She couldn't function. It wasn't the flu—this was something else.

There were no answers. Tara saw neurologists, ear, nose, and throat doctors (ENTs)—all kinds of specialists. They had nothing. No answers. Then, finally, after about six months of going through all of this, they sent her to see an infectious disease specialist, who was able to figure out the presence of Epstein-Barr virus (EBV) in Tara's body. Somehow testing for Epstein-Barr had eluded the previous doctors. Funny—they tested for mononucleosis, which is similar, but didn't think of Epstein-Barr.

Epstein-Barr is dormant in most people's bodies and only becomes active when certain things happen. In fact, EBV isn't usually detected until one has the symptoms associated with mononucleosis. Unfortunately, there is not much one can do with EBV. There is no treatment; you just have to let the body heal on its own. This is not what Tara wanted to hear! "Sorry, this is what you have, now go back to work."[69]

How could she go back to work when she could barely function? Tara couldn't walk without help. She certainly couldn't drive! She didn't have a choice, though. She was told: "Your disability is gone. We're done with you." She had to go back to work to support her family. Since Tara couldn't drive, this was how she commuted to work: her husband drove her to one of her employees' homes, who then took her to the office. Tara worked all day, holding on to the walls when she had to walk anywhere. She did this for nine months.

---

69   Wellness, Health, Mind & Spirit Body, and Autoimmune Disorders. 2017. "Epstein-Barr Virus, Epstein-Barr Symptoms | Dr. Weil." *Drweil.Com*. https://www.drweil.com/health-wellness/body-mind-spirit/autoimmune-disorders/epstein-barr/ (accessed February 28, 2017).

Nine months? You can't make this stuff up. Two days after Tara went back to work, she found out she was pregnant. She didn't even think she could have any more children. So, in addition to the EBV running rampant in her body, Tara found herself pregnant. Anything good in her body was going to her baby.

The beginning of her EBV phase was certainly more serious than while it was winding down. At first, Tara had to have someone help her walk. Later on she could walk by herself by holding onto the walls for support. When she went out with her family, she used a wheelchair. When she went to doctor appointments, Tara had to lie down in the back seat of the car or curl up in a ball in the lowered front seat. The vertigo wouldn't allow her to sit up. She said it was agony; everything was spinning and just wouldn't stop.

Vertigo is not a disease in and of itself; it's defined as a "cluster of symptoms caused by other disorders." Both stress and inflammation can lead to vertigo.[70]

Nine months later, Tara delivered a beautiful baby girl weighing only five pounds. At the time, Tara didn't realize this, but her daughter had some toxins in her body. She carefully monitored her diet for those first few months to help cleanse any impurities from her tiny baby's body. Other than that, she was healthy and all was good. Until Tara went back to work and they let her go.

Tara laughed as she told me this: "We don't want you, you're toxic and you have to go." Obviously, that's not what

---

[70] "How to Get Rid of Vertigo – Dr. Axe." 2017. *Dr. Axe.* https://draxe.com/how-to-get-rid-of-vertigo (accessed February 28, 2017).

they said to her. There was some kind of merger going on, which was perfectly reasonable. But Tara knows the truth. Out of work and still not completely well, Tara learned to adapt. She couldn't fix the vertigo, but she learned to adapt and live with it.

This went on for years. Tara described it as walking around with the flu. Imagine having the flu for years? No thank you!

In 2014, Tara stumbled upon a nurse practitioner who worked with Lyme patients. She spent a lot of time with Tara. Not something you get with the typical doctor, unfortunately. It was a holistic approach that was simply amazing. Tara was blown away. She cried during the appointment because this woman was listening to what she was saying.

They talked through Tara's entire life history, and after some testing found out that Tara had biotoxin mold illness, or chronic inflammatory response syndrome (CIRS). This was a lightbulb moment for Tara. It made perfect sense to her because she had grown up in a moldy home; she had lived in antique farmhouses and a lake house that had a flooded foundation. She had been exposed to a lot of mold throughout her entire life. She reflected that she felt the worst when she was in those homes, the ones with mold, and she started to heal when she was elsewhere. Her body knew what to do. It was trying to do its natural detoxification process, but Tara has a gene that doesn't allow her to detox properly.

With this diagnosis came a new medication called WelChol, which is technically prescribed for lowering cholesterol. It's in what pharmaceutical companies call the bile acid-binding resin class. This means it removes bile acid from the liver, so for Tara it was prescribed because it attaches to the bile (and any mold cells embedded there) that's secreted from the gall bladder and helps the body detox by releasing it as waste. She took this for about two years. She described feeling better, but not significantly. Not enough.

By this time, Tara was in a new job that was incredibly stressful and she was traveling to India frequently. Since India is on the other side of the world, she was working odd hours and had conference calls in the middle of the night. As you can imagine, this takes a toll on one's body. The first time she traveled to India was rough. The second time, about six months later, was even worse.

In 2015 she was in the middle of "the project from hell." It was an aggressive hands-on project that required more attention than anyone could give in a twenty-four-hour day. She was starting to feel weak and had a lot of pain on her left side, which is common with her illness. The pain was getting worse. She had incredible headaches, twitching in her eye, and her hands would release their grip on things. This would happen randomly. Tara would be walking around the office with a mug of tea and it would suddenly just fall out of her hands.

Doctors were recommending she go on a low- or no-amylose diet, which is like a low-carb diet except, other than bananas, fruits are allowed. It included meats, fish, poultry, eggs, dairy, nuts, and all above-ground vegetables. Essentially, this diet eliminates foods that contain "amylose and glucose which in turn cause a rapid rise in blood sugar when ingested."[71]

---

71   "No-Amylose Diet | Surviving Mold Illness." 2017. *Survivingmoldillness.Com.* http://www.survivingmoldillness.com/no-amylose-diet (accessed February 28, 2017).

Besides recommending this particular diet, doctors were telling her she needed to eat meats and bone broth. Tara is borderline-vegan and at a loss as to what to do. There weren't many options left, and she needed more than the tiny speck of food allowed to survive. She turned to a health coach, a friend from high school, to help her navigate all of this. Her coach did toxicology testing and helped Tara through an elimination diet. She worked with Tara and helped her figure out what she could eat so that Tara had some options.

Most doctors are very restrictive and will tell you what you can't have. Tara had no one telling her what she could have. Her coach helped Tara figure out what she could eat and introduced her to essential oils, which were huge in her recovery. The ball rapidly started rolling from there. Tara realized that she was getting much more out of her new diet and use of essential oils than she was from the synthetic drug she was taking.

In the back of her mind was also the crappy project she was still working on and all the added stress that entailed. She kept thinking, in July this project will be done and I'll be able to take a break. She focused on the possibility of some vacation. That didn't happen. In July there was another big project that needed Tara's skills. Tara's body didn't agree.

She doesn't remember much of July through September 2015. She doesn't remember driving to or from work. Tara only remembers working a lot, coming home, and then collapsing on the couch. Her husband took care of everything. One day in September she didn't even make it out of her car.

She remembered pulling into the driveway and just sitting there. Tara couldn't move. She felt her body melting into the seat of the car. Her husband came out after a while, wondering, what is she still doing in the car? Maybe she's on a call?

Her husband had to literally carry her inside the house. Tara went back to the doctor, who told her, "You need to make a choice. You either get better by staying home and resting and listening to your body or you go back to work and get even sicker and end up hospitalized." Tara didn't go back to work, at least not right away. There wasn't much of a choice.

Tara spent an entire week in bed thinking and recovering and trying to keep her body from shutting down. At this point, she enrolled in the Health Coach Training Program at the Institute for Integrative Nutrition (IIN) to learn more about how to take care of herself. Tara's goal was to be the healthiest version of herself that she could be. She finally left her job, for good, in May 2016 and graduated from IIN in September 2016.

Part of Tara's underlying problem was that there was mold in her house, which they were in the process of remediating. They dug up all the carpeting and put down pine flooring and cleaned up a bunch of other areas. It was a beautiful home—it just had mold in it, like most homes do. Unfortunately, Tara wasn't getting any better even after all these changes, so they made the decision to sell their home and leave. Then began the process of trying to find a home that was clean and new, that they could live in and that would help Tara move past the plateau in her healing journey.

In July 2016 they found an apartment that was brand new and had never been lived in. So the only thing Tara was subjected to was the off-gassing from the newness of the building. Within a month in their new home, Tara felt amazing. It was so different. She had removed herself from the mold; she was finishing the program at IIN and making so many changes to her health and what she was putting into her body. She was eating the right foods that were helping her. Even more so was how she was treating her body. She no longer had the stress from her job. She was taking the time to do the things she needed to do for her health and well-being. And she was resting! There were other things as well, but all these things that Tara listed, in her opinion, made a huge difference in her quality of life.

She went from not being able to find words, not being able to walk without holding onto a wall, feeling dizzy and sick, having pain all over her body—to having pain-free days. Tara no longer has vertigo, she isn't searching for words as much, and her brain fog continues to improve. She described the difference as like night and day, by making these changes and listening to her body.

She's removed lots of toxins from her home and from her life, which has also made a huge difference. It's allowed her body to return to its natural functioning, where it is detoxing on its own. Tara's body was so overloaded before that it couldn't function; it couldn't get rid of the mold. There were so many toxins coming from so many directions.

Today, Tara is an IIN graduate and she said this literally changed her life. Working with a health coach piqued her curiosity and set her on the path. But, being in the school herself and learning how important it is to listen to your body's messages, learning to take the time for rest and self-love and self-care changed everything. She can never go back to working a corporate job. Never. That kind of lifestyle no longer makes sense to her.

Being a health coach is something she can do at home. She can have a career and rest when she needs to. She can work her health-coaching business around a schedule that makes sense to her. She can be there with and for her children whenever they need her and whenever she wants.

Invariably, once or twice a month, Tara will enter a building that has mold in it and it makes her sick. Before, she would be out of work for a week or two. This severely limited where she went because there were so few places she thought were safe. If she didn't think it was safe, it was too much of a risk to her health. If she enters a moldy building now, she is knocked out for the day, or two at most. Not two weeks. With her new lifestyle, one or two days is not so bad. She can work around this. Her schedule is on her terms.

This is how Tara gauges her recovery: how quickly she bounces back from exposure to mold. Along with her blood work, of course. But she now knows how to listen to her body. When she does have an exposure, her body is able to recover much more quickly than in the past. She also has a protocol to follow when this happens and it helps her immensely.

Tara is so incredibly happy that she feels so much better. She can enjoy her family. She enjoys life again! How many people in the world today aren't like this? Questions like this get Tara's wheels turning. She can't keep this to herself. In November 2015, Tara officially started her business Be Vibrant Living. It's still a work-in-progress, but she's got some office space and she's starting to do some workshops on toxins, essential oils, and healthy eating. She said: "It feels so good. It's work that doesn't feel like work." She gets up in the morning and is excited to do this! How many people get to say that?

She has knowledge that she feels the need to share. For example, if people in the grocery store look confused, Tara will go up to them and ask if they need help. This need to share is not an obligation, though. It's more of an "Oh my gosh, I want to educate the world so that they can be healthier and happier too."

There is no one in Tara's family that has been officially diagnosed with biotoxin mold illness or CIRS, but she has suspicions about some of her siblings. Unfortunately, they have a different philosophy when it comes to health and wellness. They continue to see specialists who can't seem to diagnose their issues correctly. Tara tells them to get tested. It is genetic. But they don't listen.

Her father passed away when Tara was seventeen—from leukemia, which is also a blood disorder. According to Tara, there is some linkage between mold illness and leukemia and the weakness that her dad had. He had all kinds of health issues and challenges. Tara thinks it came from his side of the family, mainly because her mom has lived in a moldy house most of her life and still does. Her mom is perfectly fine and has no issues with mold. Also, Tara's siblings from her dad show similar symptoms, whereas her mother's child does not. Tara can tell that a few of her relatives have it, but they're not getting diagnosed and they're not helping themselves.

With her mom, Tara tried to approach it a different way. She won't listen to some of what Tara has to say, but if she says it differently her mom pays attention. For example, saying something like, "You know eating organic and making sure your food choices are non-GMO is what you used to do without having to put a label on it. This is what your parents did. Back a few decades, we didn't have to worry about food being certified as organic or non-GMO." Saying it that way made sense to Tara's mom. Fortunately, she's seventy-five and healthy as a horse.

Sadly, Tara can never go into her childhood home again, the home in which her mom lives. When her mom comes to visit Tara, there is a complicated protocol she has to go through to ensure Tara doesn't get sick from any mold spores she may be carrying. She has to shower first thing in the morning; wash and dry her clothes; put them on and then get in her car to drive to Tara's. Once she arrives, she has to go directly to the deck outside and take everything off and put something else on. Something that was washed at Tara's home that never left the premises. Every time she visits.

If her mom doesn't do all of this, Tara gets sick. For the first couple of years, Tara couldn't muster up the courage to say anything to her mom, so she suffered. One Christmas, Tara's mom came and, of course, had presents for everyone, bags of clothes, etc. Tara had to leave the room almost immediately.

Her chest got congested. It was overwhelming and she literally had to go outside her home to breathe. She didn't want her kids to miss out on Christmas with their grandmother, so Tara left.

It was after that incident that Tara had a real heart-to-heart talk with her mom. She had to explain what happened and said there have to be some rules. This was her house, and it took her a couple of days to get it back to where she needed it to be. She was sick for days. At Christmas. This conversation with her mom was a long time coming and extremely difficult. Her mom didn't understand, but Tara had to tell her, "If you don't do these things—you can't come to my house." She had to tell her mom, "I can never go to your house again and I can never sit in your car." Tara explained to me that "never, never, never, no no no" was all that was coming out of her mouth. She had to find a way to turn that around and say, "well let's do this instead." This is where they came up with a protocol for her mom to visit. That coupled with Tara using air purifiers and opening all the windows made it tolerable.

Tara told me towards the end of our conversation that the best thing she ever did for herself was go through the program at IIN. Regardless of the tests, doctors, diagnoses, she said, "I honestly in my heart of hearts believe I am healthy today because of what I learned about listening to my body." This program is life changing.

Inspiration:

Tara's journey in regaining her health taught her some incredible lessons about life, love, happiness, and self-determination. Prior to this, she had it all wrong. Now she feels that she is making it right—she's on the right path and she has a purpose. She knows that she doesn't need a corporate career, title, or anything material to define her. She is brave and strong and beautiful. It's when everything is silent that Tara hears the loudest, for she is her own biggest advocate and her voice will be heard. She has so much passion for health and wellness, and her mission is to share it with everyone who will listen.

When her symptoms were at their worst, Tara kept thinking of ways to adapt to her situation. She developed everyday survival skills that kept her motivated. She knew that there was something very wrong with her and she never, ever gave up. If no one listened, she spoke louder or found a different approach. She knew she would find her answers. She knew the universe would provide her the answers she needed to understand what was wrong and why she was chosen for this path. Now she knows and she can share her knowledge with others.

Advice:

First and foremost, don't ever give up! There is so much beauty in the world to explore. Always have faith in yourself. Get lots of fresh air and move even the smallest bit more. When you listen to what your body is trying to tell you, the path will start to reveal itself. It may be a bit of trial and error along with research but please, please, please don't ever give up. Find someone that will honestly listen to you and your symptoms. Find a Health Coach.

Contact information:

Today, Tara is a Certified Holistic Health Coach and Certified Detox Specialist, eager to speak with you about your specific health and wellness goals. If you'd like more information or would like to work with or contact Tara, check out her website: www.bevibrantliving.com

Chapter 10

Noelle: Mononucleosis and Epstein-Barr Virus

*The art of medicine consists of amusing the
patient while nature cures the disease.*

—Voltaire

Noelle

In her early twenties, Noelle came down with something her doctors couldn't diagnose. Repeated visits resulted in different possibilities. It was an upper respiratory infection, then it was strep throat, then it was something else. Each visit led to a different medication to try to clear up whatever was going on, but the combination of all these medications led to complications and ultimately a downward spiral. Her body was so out of whack, as she put it, and failing. She had a kidney infection from overuse of antibiotics, so they put her on a stronger one, which she ended up being highly allergic to. This required a Benadryl shot to counter the allergic reaction as well as a steroid. Then she was anemic, meaning her iron count was low, so they gave her iron supplements. She wondered, how does your body go from not feeling well to feeling absolutely horrible, and they don't even have a prognosis? They couldn't put a name to what was wrong with her! She was a hot mess.

This back and forth went on for a couple of years. Noelle never felt like herself. She was constantly sick. As it turned out, Noelle had had mononucleosis, common among teens and young adults. Mononucleosis—mono for short—develops from the Epstein-Barr virus, which almost everyone carries. It's an infectious disease that typically results in a sore throat, fever, swollen lymph glands, and fatigue.[72] For Noelle, it got to where she just couldn't stand it anymore and decided to start doing her own research. She wanted a more holistic approach to self-care and stopped going to doctors. If they weren't going to help her get better, she was going to take things into her own hands. They never gave her the information she needed, such as interaction of medications and other supplements. It was always "here, just take this and we'll check back with you in a couple of weeks." To quote a cliché, Noelle was sick and tired of being sick and tired.

Initially, Noelle did things like drinking more water and moving her body more. These may sound simple, but they have a huge impact. Just adding more water into your day helps to improve alertness, digestion, skin, joint lubrication,

---

72 Wellness, Health, Mind & Spirit Body, and Autoimmune Disorders. 2017. "Epstein-Barr Virus, Epstein-Barr Symptoms | Dr. Weil." *Drweil.Com.* https://www.drweil.com/health-wellness/body-mind-spirit/autoimmune-disorders/epstein-barr/ (accessed March 15, 2017).

blood, bones, and detoxification. Think about this: our bodies are approximately 63% water; our brain 75%, blood 80%, and bones are about 50% water. Water is life.[73]

Additional changes included her diet and eliminating those "quick fix" items like vitamins and pills. Noelle said this took some time, but eventually her body began to heal. She noted it mostly came down to awareness. A close friend at the time, Devynn, helped her through this period. Noelle said he should have been a health coach. He knew things instinctively, without ever studying. He would tell her things like, "Why don't you just get out. Breathe fresh air. Drink more. Eat better." She laughed at first, thinking that's not going to help. Her body wasn't working and the doctors couldn't figure it out, so how are these things going to help me? Devynn told her, "Stop stressing, drink some water, and then go for a walk after that." He was right. She needed a reset, time to heal, time to be with nature, and time to reconsider her lifestyle choices. It was eye opening to say the least. Devynn was her accountability partner long before she knew what that meant. He kicked her butt every day and kept her on track towards healing. She is forever grateful to him for the care and compassion he showed her at a time when she needed it the most. Care and compassion, by the way, that she never received from her primary care provider.

Devynn also lent her some books to keep her occupied, such as *The Secret*. Noelle began to realize that you shouldn't blindly believe everything you're told. You have to think about

---

73 "The Dr. Weil Blog – Best in Health, Fitness, Recipes, & Natural Remedies." 2017. *Drweil.Com*. http://www.drweilblog.com/home/2012/9/24/6-reasons-to-drink-water.html (accessed March 15, 2017).

and focus on what you want yourself and your life to be. It's all about the Laws of Attraction. In other words, if you want health—you must think healthy and positive thoughts. What you think about comes about, so if you focus on "why am I sick?" or "I don't want to be sick," the universe hears "sick" and that's what you get. If you focus your thoughts on health, healthy living, being vibrant and strong—that's what you attract and that's what you get more of.

She started doing things that were natural, listening to her body and taking care of herself more. She paid attention to what her body was trying to tell her. Noelle said, "There is no magic thing about this; it's about self-care." She stopped taking supplements; she stopped eating sugar; she stopped eating a lot of meat; she added more water to her day; she eliminated heavy bulky stuff like pasta and pastries. All the junk she grew up on was now out of her diet, and she started to feel a lot better. This change helped Noelle a lot. She didn't realize how sluggish she had become, and changing her diet in this way transformed her from the inside out. It's funny how a little bit of tweaking your diet and a little bit of lifestyle changes and commitment help on so many levels!

About a year and a half ago, Noelle tried the candida diet. Candida is yeast overgrowth that occurs in the digestive tract (and other places), where bad gut bacteria overpower the good gut bacteria. This is caused by many factors including too many antibiotics. Whether you have candida or simply want to heal your gut, this diet will help. Basically it calls for eliminating or at least greatly reducing things like sugar and processed foods; beer and wine; fruit and juices; gluten and wheat; beans, legumes, and starchy vegetables; and sometimes dairy.[74]

Her husband, Gene, was having a difficult time with carbs where he would get overly drowsy, had frequent infections, brain fog, some sexual issues, etc. They did some research and candida toxicity seemed fitting for his symptoms. To be supportive, Noelle did the candida diet with him. It was difficult for her because the diet seemed very limiting, and she almost gave up two weeks in. At this point, though, Gene was going through detox symptoms, and she stuck with it to help him through.

With any change in diet, especially a drastic change, you are going to experience detox symptoms. This means that your body is eliminating toxins—from your liver, kidneys, lymphatic system, bowels, skin, etc.—and while it's doing that, you have this toxic trash traveling throughout your body. Thus, you may feel things like headaches, fatigue, cravings, aches and pain, stomach issues, irritability, etc. According to Dr. Hyman, "Initially feeling bad is a good thing. It means you're on the way to getting clean."[75]

After following this diet for a while, Gene felt amazing and all of his issues went away. Noelle felt an improvement, but she didn't have as many of the same issues to begin with so the diet didn't have as big an impact on her as it did on Gene. With this experience, though, Noelle learned that limiting

74 MD, Amy. 2017. "9 Foods to Ditch If You Have Candida – Amy Myers MD." *Amy Myers MD.* http://www.amymyersmd.com/2016/07/9-foods-to-avoid-if-you-have-candida/ (accessed March 15, 2017).

75 2017. http://drhyman.com/blog/2016/05/12/8-tips-to-ease-detox-discomfort/retrieved (accessed March 15, 2017).

carbs and sugars was good for her. She knows that when she does ingest these things, she feels "icky." She is definitely glad she tried it.

Growing up in a traditional Italian family means huge family-style meals—feasts, really, with lots of heavy pasta, breads, meat sauces, pastries, etc. Every morning for Noelle was like Sunday morning to the rest of us: coffee and pastries. Carbs and sugars were ingrained in her. It's how she grew up. They were a part of who she was, and changing her diet and lifestyle meant giving up a part of her past. Giving up a piece of herself. She knew something had to change, though, so she pushed through her fears and decided to trust that the universe had her back and that change was good.

Noelle reflected that her mom wasn't into all the traditional Italian foods, but she felt it was the most nutritious food to give her two daughters. She would say things like, "I don't eat a lot of red meat but I know you guys need the protein." They also had vegetables and fruits, but these were minimal. The focus was on bulk, as Noelle put it.

It was a difficult transition, changing her diet so much and turning down foods she frequently ate in the past. At the time she had three jobs and had been guzzling coffee all day. It was totally unhealthy. Trying to stop all of these unhealthy things at once brought on symptoms of detox, as mentioned earlier. Noelle described the way she had been feeling as "crash and burn, all the time." She had headaches, jitters, and dehydration. What made it even more difficult was that her family didn't understand. They would say things like, "What do you mean you don't want pizza?" And when she told them, "Don't buy Twinkies, I'm not going to eat them," they would respond with, "Why, what's wrong with you?" Noelle wasn't trying to be insulting to her family, but she knew she couldn't eat the same way she always had. She needed to be healthy.

This change took time. It didn't happen overnight. Noelle told me it took about two years to make the changes to her diet, and that it didn't really stick until about year five. It took five years for her to get it where it was now a habit and didn't require much thought. Going through the Health Coach Training Program at the Institute for Integrative Nutrition confirmed for her that she was on the right track. Everything she learned at IIN validated all the changes she had already made in her diet and lifestyle.

It wasn't five solid years of change. As with most things in life, it takes time for habits to form and for us humans to learn new ways. For Noelle, it was on and off. It took years for her body to heal and she still felt terrible, but she was determined. She started purchasing some of the household groceries back when she was still with her parents and would make healthy substitutions. For example, she would buy ground turkey in-stead of ground beef. She still made their traditional Italian dishes that everyone liked, but she made them healthier.

This was a big deal for Noelle; as mentioned earlier, her Italian heritage meant a lot to her. It was a big part of who she was, but she learned that you don't have to give up tradition or the things you love for a diet change. There are ways to keep those traditions alive by finding healthier ways of cooking traditional foods.

It's interesting that Noelle thought she used to complain a lot about her condition when she was feeling awful for years. Personally, I feel it's your right to complain about not feeling well—especially if it goes on for years and you don't have an answer! She reflected that she didn't have a major problem; rather it was something that could have been prevented or "fixed" earlier if she had been diagnosed properly and if she had received guidance from her primary caregivers about nutrition and things like water and sleep. There is a gap there; there's something missing when doctors don't tell you the nutritional aspect of health, when they don't look at the whole person and that person's lifestyle. Instead, the general trend seems to be that you go back to the practice and see a totally different person who has never seen you before, whom you will never see again. It doesn't make sense.

These days Noelle prefers functional medicine specialists who look at the whole person. When she was pregnant she decided not to have a traditional obstetrician. She did at first, but she never saw the same person twice and they never spent more than five minutes with her. She wanted a relationship with the medical professional who would be taking care of her through the nine months of pregnancy. She wanted consistency, someone who knew her medical history so she didn't have to repeat it every time. So, Noelle started seeing two midwives who stayed with her throughout her entire pregnancy. She loved them and they never left her side.

After Noelle's daughter was born, she experienced the

same thing with her pediatrician. The baby had diaper rash, and Noelle took her to a doctor who prescribed a cream for her. That didn't work, so she went back and they gave her something even stronger. That didn't help either. Noelle was at a loss. She was frazzled and in anguish hearing her child screaming in pain. She finally searched online for "natural remedies for diaper rash" and found a woman who used plain, unsweetened Greek yogurt. It may sound weird, but it totally healed the diaper rash. Noelle put the cold yogurt on her daughter's rear and the next day all was well. There must be something about the cultures in the yogurt that attack the yeast in the diaper rash. Fascinating! The $50 cream prescribed by the doctor did nothing, and the $3 yogurt from the supermarket healed her. That was another example to Noelle that she is on the right path. A path that she is determined to share with others.

Inspiration:

Going through her journey put Noelle on track to become a health coach. It solidified her understanding that there is a gap between the patient and doctor and basic things like diet and self-care. As a health coach, she can be that bridge—to prevent, to guide, and to create awareness. While she was going through her misdiagnosis, Noelle's grandmother became ill with colon cancer. This was a huge shock as there was no family history of cancer. This became part of Noelle's story that she wanted to share. Noelle said that if she can help even just one person, she is content. She wants to spread awareness.

She wants her story to offer hope and an understanding that there can be a different way.

Advice:

When you're in your darkest moments, write down what you're feeling. Journal it. Then go back the next day and read it over. Feel it. Immerse yourself in it. See if there are any adjustments you can make. Try something to bring you a little closer to your goal. Understand that there is always another way. Even if/when you feel the absolute worst, don't take one person's opinion. Seek out another option. Keep reaching out. Try to see a different outcome. There is always more than what you see and what you are feeling. There is always hope. If you have hope, you have health.

Contact:

Noelle is a graduate of the Institute for Integrative Nutrition's Health Coach Training Program and is inspired to spread awareness about holistic approaches to health and wellness. If you've been touched by Noelle's story and want to work with her or contact her, she can be found at her blog site: https://girlredesigned.wordpress.com/

Chapter 11

Denise: Genetic Migraines

Every time you eat or drink, you are either
feeding disease or fighting it.

—Anonymous

Denise

Approximately four years ago, Denise was struggling in her daily life with extremely low energy, very bad migraines, and stomach issues. She said she felt exhausted—all the time, every day.

She had been suffering for a while and didn't know what, if anything, she could do. Fortunately, a high school friend invited her over for lunch. But it was a very different lunch than what Denise had been expecting. Her friend was having a meal-replacement shake. Denise asked her about it, and they had a long conversation about this amazing nutrient-dense superfood program with shakes and nutritional cleansing and adaptogens. If this sounds familiar, it's the same program that Nicole used to get her life back.

Denise wasn't even thinking about how bad she felt. She wasn't thinking this could help her migraines. Why would she think food could help? Wouldn't her doctors have mentioned that? All she heard was that it helped with weight loss, so Denise thought, okay, cool, I would love to lose about ten pounds so let me try this. She had no idea that this program to help her release some weight would help relieve her suffering as well.

This particular nutritional cleansing program has systems for energy, performance, healthy aging, and, of course, weight loss. The protocol for the weight loss system means replacing two meals per day with their meal-replacement shakes. These are not your typical protein shakes. They are in fact "meal replacement" shakes consisting of 24 grams of both protein and carbohydrates as well as five grams of fat and eight grams of fiber. Enough to keep you satiated for a few hours. Denise replaced her breakfast and lunch with the shakes and then had dinner with her family: a healthy 400–600 calorie dinner. The protocol also recommends healthy snacks, or about 100–150 calories between meals, to keep your metabolism up.

Her days now started with a 2-ounce shot of an herbal tonic infused with minerals, vitamins, nutrients, and plant-based adaptogens, all of which are designed to help manage stress and fatigue. There was also a "cleanse"—and not the kind that has you in the bathroom all day long. This particular cleanse, made with herbs and botanicals, helps support the body's natural filters to enhance detoxification at the cellular level. It also boosts metabolism and energy, protects cells and vital organs from aging, and increases mental clarity. Who couldn't use more of that! The cleanse can be done in a number of different ways, including an all-day cleanse (up to two consecutive days) or daily, taken first thing in the morning.

After about a week of using these products, Denise realized that she felt better. She told me she felt tremendous relief from all the ailments she listed above, specifically the headaches and the stomach issues. She also had more energy, was sleeping more soundly, was in a better mood, and she felt happier. Let me repeat that: she was happier! She loved the way she felt.

From that moment on, Denise knew she would never be without these products in her body. Over the next few months, her migraines continued to decrease in frequency and they were more manageable. Four years later, she still feels the same. Amazing. Healthy. Happy. Energetic.

Before beginning her nutritional cleansing program, Denise's diet was not the greatest. She told me she didn't eat all that much and wasn't getting enough calories in her daily routine. Though at the time she thought what she was eating was okay. It wasn't like she was feeding her family fast food every night. Looking back, though, now that she knows more about nutrition, minerals, vitamins, botanicals, etc., Denise understands she wasn't eating as well as she could have.

Her breakfast staples included things like dry cereals, English muffins, corn muffins, yogurt, and coffee, etc. Not the most nutritious foods. Denise never paid much attention to what she was eating or the ingredients with which she cooked. The truth is she didn't know what or how to eat. Family dinners included things like steaks, sausage and peppers, hamburgers, chicken parmesan, and a lot of pasta. Yes, they're Italian. She still makes chicken parmesan, for example, but uses better oils and cheeses and the chicken is organic and free-range. They've also cut down on their beef intake and eat much more chicken as well as more vegetables and salads. Overall, Denise makes better choices in the quality of the food she feeds her family. She pays very careful attention to everything, including the kinds of oils, salt, and butter she uses. She transformed the way she eats and the way she cooks for her family.

When Denise was having frequent migraines, her emotional state was in the toilet. She felt horrible. She was never in a good mood. She either had a headache and had to live with that, or she was dealing with the consequences of all the medication she had to take. Her options were simple: deal with the debilitating pain and the nausea and the light sensitivity of the migraine, or feel tired and miserable from all the medication. It was a vicious cycle. She was never well and she was not happy. *Denise never had a day where she felt good.*

Imagine the impact on your life being in constant pain, being miserable all the time. Imagine the impact on your family.

Once she changed her diet and began this program, Denise had more good days than bad. That is huge! It changed her whole life. Denise is now happy and upbeat and energetic.

She can do things every day. The things you and I take for granted. She doesn't spend her days lying down or just wanting to sleep. She is active and out and about.

When Denise was suffering with horrible migraines, she often called her mom to come over and watch the kids while she rested. Or she would have to call her husband, who would have to stop what he was doing and come home from work, or pick up the kids from school, or whatever had to be done. Denise could not do it so someone else had to. She couldn't drive in that painful state. She could barely function. This impacted everyone. Her entire family. Even her kids. Especially her kids.

Her husband, Steven, came home to help her—happily, though at times it was difficult since he was running a landscaping business and was stressed. Imagine your spouse in that much pain, so miserable that he or she could barely function, and at the same time you are the boss running a business that required you to be there. He was pulled in multiple directions. Worried about Denise. Worried about whatever job he was doing at the moment. Worried about leaving a worksite to go home. Worried about his business. Worried about the kids. Worried about the kids seeing Denise this way. Worry upon worry upon worry. That's no way to go through life.

Fortunately, he worked somewhat locally so he could go home. Then when Denise felt a little better, he would go back and try to finish the job. The whole time worried about his wife. Then there were times he just couldn't get home. Imagine the guilt he felt!

Early on in their relationship, Denise wasn't yet on the correct prescription. It wasn't strong enough. She would take it, but her migraine would not go away. One night Steven brought her to their first house he had purchased right before they got married. He was living there while doing work on the house, but she was not yet living there. Denise was so sick they had to stay the night. That's the first time Steven really saw how bad it could be. Denise was miserable, in pain, and crying. Thinking back, she reflected that she should have gone to the emergency room that night. But she didn't. She tried to ride it out.

Halfway into our interview, Denise told me she has had migraines since she was five years old. *Five* years old! She would get sent home from school once or twice per week—sometimes more. Every week. Back then they didn't have the kinds of medication we have today. They gave her codeine because that was the only thing that helped even a little. She would go to sleep until she was better. There was nothing else you could do back then.

Denise told me the codeine didn't make the migraine go away, it only took the edge off. That's it. So for a day or two, she would live with this pain until the migraine finally ran its course and went away on its own.

Now at least she has better medication so on the rare occasions she gets a migraine, she takes her medication and it's gone in an hour. That's it. An hour. So she never has to live through that pain and the associated symptoms anymore. Denise still might get one or two migraines per month, but in the past it was sixteen every month. Think about that. That's four migraines every week!

According to the Mayo Clinic, "a migraine can cause se-vere throbbing pain or a pulsing sensation, usually on just one side of the head. It's often accompanied by nausea, vomiting, and extreme sensitivity to light and sound."[76] Migraines last for many hours and sometimes even days. The pain can be debilitating. Denise didn't simply have migraines. She had *chronic* migraines. This meant that she had severe headaches fifteen or more days per month, and each headache lasted four or more hours. It also meant that at least eight of those fifteen headaches were migraines.[77] It's no wonder Denise is thrilled to have found this nutritional cleansing system. It has changed her life.

Along with their nutritional cleansing program, Denise and her husband completely changed the way they eat. As much as possible they choose organic, grass-fed, free-range, fresh, whole, non-processed foods, etc. They do chicken a lot of different ways. Sometimes with sautéed vegetables, some-times like a cutlet, sometimes grilled. They no longer eat sau-sage and peppers or steaks, and only eat hamburgers once in a while. Even dairy is mostly gone from their house with only some organic cream for coffee. The quality of what they put in and even on their bodies has improved greatly.

As for her three kids, they have added some of the nutri-tional products into their regimen, such as the shakes and bars. They still love eggs, though, so Denise buys free-range

76 2017. http://www.mayoclinic.org/diseases-conditions/migraine-headache/home/ovc-20202432 (accessed January 30, 2017).
77 "Chronic Migraine by the Numbers." 2017. *My Chronic Migraine.* https://www.mychron-icmigraine.com/living-with-chronic-migraine?cid=sem_goo_43700007344044820 (accessed January 30, 2017).

eggs for them to make scrambled eggs or French toast. Her oldest daughter now asks for a shake in the mornings. She also suffers from headaches, and she realized that when she has the meal-replacement shakes on a regular basis, she feels better. Denise told me in a later conversation that her mom and her grandmother both had severe migraines as well. So apparently it runs in her family, at least on the female side.

Denise was five when she started having migraines; her mother was eleven; her grandmother was in her early teens; and her oldest daughter was a teenager as well when her migraines began. According to Dr. Richard Pearl, a clinical neurologist, "a combination of genetics and environment play a role" in migraine headaches.[78] This is definitely the case with Denise's family.

Nutrition is key. Denise never knew this before. She never understood how important it is for your body to eat the right things and in the right amounts. For example, for breakfast Denise used to eat nutritionally bankrupt foods like corn muffins and coffee. Her husband would eat a bagel with cream cheese or a ham, egg, and cheese sandwich and coffee. That's completely changed. They both begin their day with a shot of cleanse, a shot of adaptogenic tonic, their nutrient-dense meal-replacement shakes, and their vitamins. She loves this system and how easy it is for her to do every day. It's convenient, easy, and portable; all you have to do is add water and shake it up.

78 "Are Migraines Hereditary?" 2017. *Migrainehelper.Com.* http://www.migrainehelper.com/migraine-occurrence-in-women-and-families.shtml (accessed April 5, 2017).

Inspiration:

The right nutrition can change everything. Organic foods and supplements rule supreme. Denise never realized how significant what you feed your body on a daily basis is. Food puts your body in balance—or not. When it's not in balance, you're sick in some way. Whether it's with migraines or something else, just changing your nutrition is so worth it. For Denise, finding out, after all that time, that there was an answer to help her was huge. She thought she would spend her entire life having migraines and feeling miserable. Now she enjoys life. This is so powerful—that nutrition can change everything, *even genetic predispositions.*

Advice:

Denise advises us to cleanse our bodies and change our nutrition. Sure, you can live with migraines and know that eventually the pain will be gone. You know there's going to be a time when you can function again. But why suffer when you can change your diet and feel amazing?

Contact:

If you suffer from migraines and want more information or simply want to work with Denise towards a better diet and lifestyle, you can call her at 973-819-0299, or send her an e-mail at Lucca2000@optonline.net

PART FOUR

Illnesses
Surfacing On
The Skin

Chapter 12

When Your Skin Tells You What Is Really Going On Inside Your Body

When we talk about the world we live in today with pollutants affecting our air, our water, our oceans, our food, what part of our lives is unaffected? And which is the largest organ of the body that is increasingly showing the impact of our bad behaviors? It is without a doubt, our skin.

The leading affliction and illness on the rise today is psoriasis. According to the National Psoriasis Foundation, not only is psoriasis the most prevalent autoimmune disease in the United States, but "there are as many as 7.5 million Americans—approximately 2.2% of the population—who suffer from psoriasis,"[79] and, according to the World Psoriasis Day consortium 125 million people worldwide—2% to 3% of the total population. Once again, the numbers are absolutely staggering.

---

79   2017. http://ttp://www.mg217.com/your-psoriasis/statistics-about-psoriasis/ (accessed February 20, 2017).

The red patchy, thick scales that form on the skin have eluded physicians, and 20 to 30 percent of people end up with psoriatic arthritis, which is even more painful and debilitating than psoriasis itself. Just to keep you informed, according to the medical community (and even the National Psoriasis Foundation) there is no cure.

Another illness that often presents through the skin, other than the common ones we hear about like eczema and acne which are not labeled autoimmune, is a less-well-known illness called lupus. Lupus often presents with a butterfly-type rash over the nose and cheeks. Both of these are believed to be genetic.

For psoriasis, according to psoriasis.org, "Scientists have now identified about 25 genetic variants that make a person more likely to develop psoriatic disease. At the University of Michigan, Dr. J.T. Elder and his team of researchers have identified several areas on the human genome where more than one gene may be involved in psoriasis and psoriatic arthritis." As a matter of fact, "At the University of California–San Francisco, Dr. Wilson Liao is using new genetic sequencing technology to find rare 'trigger genes' that may be the leading causes of psoriasis in certain individuals."[80]

An interesting article entitled "What does heredity have to do with it?" said:

Scientists now believe that at least 10 percent of the general population inherits one or more of the genes

<hr>

[80] "Science of Psoriasis: Genes and Psoriatic Disease | National Psoriasis Foundation." 2017. *Psoriasis.Org*. https://www.psoriasis.org/research/genes-and-psoriatic-disease (accessed February 20, 2017).

that create a predisposition to psoriasis. However, only two percent to three percent of the population develops the disease.

This is thought to be because only two percent to three percent of people encounter the "right" mix of genetics and are exposed to triggers that lead to the development of psoriasis. Those who have a genetic disease but don't have a family history of it, for example, may have inherited two genes from their father and two from their mother—neither of whom had all four and therefore never developed the disease.

Working with DNA samples from a large family that includes many people with psoriasis, Anne Bowcock, Ph.D., a professor of genetics at Washington University School of Medicine in St. Louis, has identified a gene mutation known as CARD14 that when activated with an environmental trigger leads to plaque psoriasis.

Therefore this article confirms everything that I have been saying, which is that environment is what exacerbates illnesses such as psoriasis and genetics isn't everything.

As for lupus, technically called systemic lupus erythematosus (SLE), the "word 'lupus' (from the Latin word for 'wolf') is attributed to the thirteenth century physician Rogerius, who used it to describe erosive facial lesions that were reminiscent of a wolf's bite. The word 'erythematosus' (from the Greek word 'erythros,' meaning red) refers to the reddish color of the discoid facial lesions."[81]

---

81   2017. http://www.lupus.org/answers/entry/where-did-the-name-lupus-come (accessed April 15, 2017).

Systemic lupus erythematosus (SLE) is another extremely complicated autoimmune system disease where the body attacks its own cells and the reason to the medical community is unclear, but again, there is no cure. It can affect any organ of the body and can cause joint stiffness, swelling, pain, fevers, malaise, etc. It is chronic, painful, comes and goes, and the patient truly does not know what they are up against each and every new day. This is mentally confusing, grueling, and devastating, and to keep oneself optimistic while in pain and having no idea what the outcome of your illness may be can wear even the strongest personality down.

To date there is no specific *gene* that has been declared as making lupus hereditary; however, there can be common family traits. "No gene or group of genes has been proven to cause lupus. Lupus does, however, appear in certain families, and when one of two identical twins has lupus, there is an increased chance that the other twin will also develop the disease. These findings, as well as others, strongly suggest that genes are involved in the development of lupus. Although lupus can develop in people with no family history of lupus, there are likely to be other autoimmune diseases in some family members. Certain ethnic groups (people of African, Asian, Hispanic/Latino, Native American, Native Hawaiian, or Pacific Island descent) have a greater risk of developing lupus, which may be related to genes they have in common."[82]

One of the problems that I see with both lupus and psoriasis and so many other of these illnesses is that the first mode

---

82 2017. http://www.lupus.org/answers/entry/is-lupus-hereditary (accessed April 15, 2017).

of medical treatment is usually steroids or some immunosuppressive drug. What is so scary about this is that it is those precise drugs that tend to set the patient up for extremely rough side effects, while breaking the body and immune system down so much that it leaves the patient open to deadly infections. This is why it is so important to disseminate and share these stories, because people who are on steroids for life are hurting themselves and in essence shortening their "healthy" lifespan.

Despite the genetic news and studies, finally there is awakening happening as information is being shared on how to treat psoriasis naturally and effectively, and people have shown 100% cure rates or remission where there are absolutely no lesions showing on the skin for periods of time. I am not going to spend time describing this illness because of the interview that I had with Kim Weiler, who recently published a book on the topic. Kim suffered from psoriasis for over 21 years, trying all sorts of pharmaceuticals and remedies. She certainly seems to have unlocked some mysteries and is now sharing how she has healed herself. She is another Institute for Integrative Nutrition (IIN) graduate, an internationally certified health coach, and is busy disseminating this information as you will read in her story.

One of the common results of these immune system disorders that are visible for the world to see (because the skin is screaming out, please pay attention to my innards) is this constant psychological trauma. Unfortunately, most people who see the lesions on the skin have a reaction of fear that it might be contagious. That one reaction and/or rejection by another human being can be devastating, and to walk around with this condition plays major havoc on an individual's self-esteem.

This is why no matter what, our world needs to pay attention to working through any medical illness from a 3-point view of mind-body-spirit, and as we learn at IIN, bio-individuality. Joshua Rosenthal, the founder and director of IIN, explained it like this: one person's medicine is another person's poison. "Bio-individuality means that no one diet works for everyone. Each and every person has unique needs." Essentially, there is not just one answer; there is not one thing that will work for everyone. The answers are as unique as we humans are. A cure is a special and individual process that includes everything we put in our bodies, on our bodies, and everything we feed (negatively or positively) to our spirit.[83] It is certainly okay to explore what the medical profession has to say, but to stop there would be to greatly decrease your chances of achieving optimal health and permanent healing. There is so much more that can be done than just taking steroids or using topical medications that may not even work and most likely have side effects. Don't you owe it to yourself to step up to a 3-point perspective and get healed?

83 "Joshua Rosenthal's Bio-Individuality Is Scientifically Proven." 2017. *Institute for Integrative Nutrition.* http://www.integrativenutrition.com/blog/2015/07/joshua-rosenthal-s-bio-individuality-is-scientifically-proven (accessed April 28, 2017).

Chapter 13

Kim: Psoriasis

Dogs do speak, but only to those who know how to listen.

—Orphan Pamuk

Kim

I first met Kim through e-mail when we were beginning our health coach studies at the Institute for Integrative Nutrition. Somehow a group of five of us connected and became each other's accountability partners throughout the year-long program. I'm still not quite sure how that happened, but I am grateful every day for these ladies in my life!

Kim has had psoriasis, an autoimmune chronic skin disease, since the age of nineteen; she's forty now, so that's a long time. Since that age of about nineteen, Kim's career was in the television and film industry. Looking back, she realizes that it was an incredibly stressful environment, which is significant because scientists have been learning that stress contributes to autoimmune issues.

A native New Yorker, Kim grew up on Long Island and moved to Manhattan when she was twenty-five. She had a great life. She was working in television production, her dream job, and living in the city. Kim was living her dream life in her dream city. She had *the* life. It was wonderful! But ... Kim had this secret that she always carried around with her. She did a tremendous job of covering it up, and very few people in her life knew that that secret was psoriasis.

Basically, Kim was living with a lie for half her life. No added stress there! She lied about this to most of her friends. A lie of omission. She never talked about it. She never complained or vented about it. She hid it.

On a vacation in Cancun, Mexico, with friends when she was twenty-one, Kim had a horrific outbreak and had visible psoriasis all over her legs. Imagine this: it's spring break and she's on the beach in a bathing suit with nine guys, five girls, and her legs are covered with red scaly patches. Of course, everyone was asking, "What is that?" Kim recalled only telling one very good girlfriend that it was actually psoriasis. No one else knew. She remembers saying something like, "Oh, I don't know, let's go swimming," to avoid the conversation. Kim remembers being tortured on that trip because she was so embarrassed. She also had a crush on one of the guys, so her insecurities were screaming out and she knew that he sensed something was off.

For the most part, psoriasis was her secret, and this was an early memory she has where it totally affected her social life.

Kim did everything she could to cover it up, such as always wearing long-sleeved shirts and long pants in the summer and all kinds of cover-up makeup. She would also go tanning regularly so her skin would be darker and the spots would be less noticeable. Her main problem areas were her legs and elbows, though she would often get spots all over. The spots were less noticeable to most people's eyes, but Kim saw them. She always knew they were there—on her torso, her breasts, her ears, her scalp, her butt, etc. They were all over.

At the time, Kim didn't realize that her self-esteem was completely shattered. She had little self-worth. She wasn't giving herself any self-love. She didn't know how to. She didn't even know there was such a thing.

Reflecting on her childhood, Kim said her dad was a loving father. Her mom was different. She was loving in her own way, but not in the outward affectionate way that her dad was. Kim's dad was also an alcoholic and became sober right around the time she manifested psoriasis. No coincidence there. She recognizes that her parents did the best they could do as far as giving her love. They certainly took care of her. But Kim didn't grow up with an awareness of self-love. This was a foreign concept to her. Unheard of.

When you're in your teens and early twenties, you really care about and dwell upon what other people think. Kim had very little self-esteem at this stage in her life, though from the outside, you wouldn't know this. She had a lot of friends, was a cheerleader, she got "most fun to be with" in her high school yearbook, and she managed to be in every theater production.

Kim was popular. Anyone looking in would think there was nothing wrong, that she had a great life. Even in college, she was going to school in New York City. She had an exciting life on the outside—but on the inside she never felt confident.

Obviously, Kim was a very good actress. She had a naturally happy and bubbly personality, and she used it well. It got her everywhere, but deep down she didn't feel good about herself because of her lesions.

So, she's in her twenties, working in the city, working in television, and everything is going great, but she is working her butt off! Kim was working fourteen- to sixteen-hour days. She was constantly getting sick and battling with her skin. Doctor after doctor would prescribe medication, such as steroid creams and ointments. They also suggested she get light therapy (phototherapy), but that involves a lot of time and must be consistent for it to work well. Kim didn't have the time for that. It's also expensive and insurance only covers a portion.[84]

Like many of us, Kim listened to her doctors who told her this condition was hereditary. Kim has since learned that only forty percent of people with psoriasis have family members who are also affected. She kept hearing that there was no cure for this autoimmune chronic skin disease and that she needed to find a way to relieve it with these creams and ointments they were prescribing. They also offered Kim oral medications, but the creams always seemed to do the trick. At least temporarily—never long enough. This cycle of seeing doctors,

---

84   2017. https://www.psoriasis.org/about-psoriasis/treatments/phototherapy (accessed March 4, 2017).

getting new/different creams, having them work for a while then stop, went on for years. She never thought to look at her psoriasis in any other way. Why would she? She was listening to her doctors, whom she trusted.

Dating was a big part of Kim's lie. She told me she essentially lied to every man she ever dated—some outright and some by omission. The only man she was truthful with about her psoriasis was her now-husband, Michael. Much of her dating years are a blur in this regard. Kim thinks she blocked a lot of it out. Obviously some men didn't get far enough for her to worry about them seeing her skin. Others dated Kim when her skin was in a period of being clear. There was a constant fear, though. Kim remembers feeling extremely self-conscious with men. She was so disgusted by her psoriasis and automatically projected that onto them, thinking they were going to be disgusted by it as well. She kept thinking, they're going to break up with me because they don't want to be with a girl with psoriasis. That's gross.

She has one particular memory when she was in bed with her boyfriend and she had a patch of psoriasis on her elbow. Kim did everything she could to make sure he wouldn't see it or touch it, like rolling around or moving her arm very quickly if he got close. She was terrified of his judgment: that is what she walked around with—every day. Being afraid of what other people would think. It's so crushing to your self-worth. And this is not just Kim. There are over 125 million people in the world with psoriasis, and many more with other skin conditions. Most of them are walking around with a lack of self-worth and in fear of people judging them or thinking they're contagious.

Kim wonders at times if she was afraid of other people's reactions or if she was afraid they would look at it the same way that she did. Many of her fears were probably projections, but who truly knows?

When she was thirty, Kim attained her dream of being an actor. This brought up old fears about her skin, having to dress for certain parts and wear specific clothing for whatever role she was playing. It scared her, but she didn't let that stop her. She became an actor despite her fears and did this for seven years. During this period, Kim thought this was what she was meant to do. She absolutely loved acting. She described it as being very therapeutic for her. In two years of acting school, Kim cried rivers of tears every other day. She got out so much emotion and believes a lot of it was not feeling good enough. Kim had been feeling that she was not enough her entire life.

At this time, Kim moved from TV production to TV accounting to have enough time for her acting schedule, as the accounting position was more flexible for her schedule. While she was acting, Kim remembers always having fear about flare-ups and what particular costume she would have to wear for a role. There was one horror film shot in the woods ('cause where else do you shoot a horror film?) with seven or eight people. Kim had a horrible patch of psoriasis on her shin at the time, getting bigger and bigger every day. She chose to wear long pants to cover her calves and a button-down shirt to hide her elbows. Everyone else was in shorts, tee shirts, and tank tops. It was the summer, very hot, and they were in the woods and Kim was covered up. She remembers thinking they were all comfortable in their skin. She was not. Ever.

While Kim was living her dream life, she wasn't appreciating it or feeling grateful for it either. She had this constant fear that if people knew her secret, they weren't going to love her. Then one day she realized that if she didn't love herself enough, if she had that belief—how could she expect other people to love her?

Then the life-changing event. When Kim was thirty-five, about five years ago, her dog Max was very sick. He was a rescue dog with every condition you could imagine. He had chronic bronchitis, arthritis in every part of his body, and epilepsy with seizures. He was also so overweight he could barely walk at times and couldn't get any exercise. Kim was not overfeeding him by any stretch of the imagination. She was buying super-expensive dog food, like $100 per bag. It was raw and organic, etc. She was trying everything she could to make his life better, but he kept gaining more weight.

Max was a small beagle and kept blowing up. Kim assumed it was because he could barely walk and was hardly moving. It got to where Kim was feeding him tiny amounts of food. She felt like she was starving him, but he kept gaining weight! She didn't understand what was happening. She was at a complete loss and poor Max kept getting sicker and sicker.

He was around ten at this time and they moved to a new neighborhood, which led to a new veterinarian. The vet asked Kim if she'd ever considered cooking whole foods for him. Like foods that you and I would eat. Huh? She told Kim you can buy the most expensive organic dog food, but at the end of the day, it's processed. It's leftover scraps and you don't know what's in it. If you cook for him, you know exactly what's going into his body. The vet said, "I guarantee you will see results if you do this for him."

Kim's first thought was, that sounds very time consuming and very expensive. Working in TV doesn't leave a lot of time for anything else. She barely had time to feed herself. The vet asked her if she could just be open to it. "Can you just try it? Do it for one week and see how it goes." Kim was desperate to help Max so she completely complied.

Right around this same time, Kim's friend Katie Newman published a book called *The Amazing Treat Diet for Dogs: How I Saved My Dog from Obesity*. Katie's Labrador, Hustler, was obese and unable to exercise due to severe joint issues. The book is about inspiring others to help their beloved pets. Kim read it cover to cover.

So Max's diet changed from raw organic bagged food to organic chicken, grass-fed beef, wild-caught salmon, organic vegetables, fruit, brown rice, and even hard-boiled eggs. Max would drool over this new food he was getting; he loved it so much. His weight loved it as well. He lost so much weight in a two-month period that Kim started worrying he was getting too skinny! Even the vet was saying he's losing too much weight. Kim was feeding him up to 3.5 cups of food every day so he could maintain his weight.

Let's backtrack a moment. When Kim was feeding Max a quarter of a cup of the dry organic food twice per day, he was gaining weight. When she fed him 3.5 cups of real whole food, he was at a healthy weight. That's three extra cups of food every day!

Before this new diet, Max could barely walk. Kim has three steps leading up from her apartment to the street. She would have to pick him up and carry him up those three steps. He would do his business, then wait for Kim to pick him up to go back into the apartment. In two months, Max went from barely walking to running up the stairs and down the street. He was running!

The vet was thrilled, as you can imagine. It was so rewarding to see a beloved pet come back to life. Within a six-month period Max had been weaned off all his medications. He had been on an inhaler and five other medications. No longer. After his annual check-up with blood work, the vet said his eleven-year-old insides were those of a six-month-old puppy.

Kim's mind was blown and a lightbulb went off. During Max's transformation, Kim had been doing more research on whole foods and watching health documentaries, reading books on health, etc. She started researching more about psoriasis and was finding thousands of items, YouTube videos, etc. She found a forum about psoriasis where you can talk to millions of other people who are going through similar issues. Kim couldn't believe how much information there was out there on the Internet, and wondered why it took her so long to figure this out. She couldn't understand why she hadn't done this kind of search before.

She was also finding a lot of information related to food and decided to talk to her dermatologist about it. Kim had already started to shift the way she was eating, mainly based on Max's results. If whole real foods could bring him back to being puppy-like, imagine what it might do for Kim? So at her next dermatologist appointment Kim asked about food. The doctor rolled her eyes and said there was absolutely no proof that changing your diet could improve your skin.

I have to repeat that. Kim's dermatologist told her that there is absolutely no proof that changing your diet can improve your skin.

Kim had never had the greatest relationship with her dermatologist. She said she always felt kind of stupid with the way the doctor responded to her questions. In the past, Kim had asked about dairy and sugar, but her doctor always had a similar response and was always defensive. Like the doctor was thinking, how dare you question my expertise? Perhaps she felt threatened that if Kim could figure out things for herself, she wouldn't need her dermatologist anymore.

Kim's gut was telling her she was on the right track, though, especially after everything she was reading and watching and after seeing Max's transformation. She was at an appointment with her dermatologist where they had been trying to treat a stubborn patch on Kim's leg, and the doctor said, "Why don't we try a shot of cortisone? That should do the trick."

Kim wanted to throw up. She literally thought she was going to vomit. She told the doctor, "no, that's okay," and walked out. At this point, Kim was beyond motivated to do something about her skin. She kept searching and researching and found a book by Dr. John Pagano called *Healing Psoriasis: The Natural Alternative*. She knew enough by now to eat whole foods, do the organic thing, etc., but this book focused specifically on psoriasis. This was a game-changer. Kim read the entire book within two days.

She was blown away again. Even though Kim's diet was healthier again, it wasn't helping her skin the way she had hoped. There was something she had been missing. This book opened her eyes. It answered all her questions. First, it explained what psoriasis was in a way her doctors never did, in a way that totally made sense to Kim. Basically Kim told me, when there is chronic inflammation in the body, our intestinal tract doesn't work as efficiently as it should and small particles are able to leak out of the intestines. These particles are basically toxins, which are normally sent out of the body via waste. When they get into your bloodstream, however (through the intestinal wall), the only way out is through the skin. Additionally, when you have psoriasis, your skin doesn't shed the way it does on other people, so it gets blocked and can form scales, patches, and plaque on the skin surface. Basically, Kim's skin was doing what her bowels and kidneys should have been doing—eliminating toxins and waste.

For sixteen years Kim had struggled with her self-worth and her self-esteem and herself because she didn't understand. No one had ever explained her condition in this way. There were answers out there the entire time. Kim never knew. It's so unfair to so many people that this information is available, it's out there, but no one hears it from their doctors. All they hear from their doctors is try this cream or this ointment or this other prescription medication or have a shot of cortisone.

Another thing she learned from Dr. Pagano's book was the difference between an alkaline and an acidic diet. Most Americans eat a highly acidic diet. Kim was no different. With her schedule and job, she was constantly eating on the go, grabbing whatever was quick and easy. She called it crap—donuts, bagels, dairy, sugar, lots of processed food—and though not a big drinker, she was going out for happy hour all the time, and coffee was her go-to. One category that shocked Kim was nightshade vegetables, which include, among other things, tomatoes, potatoes, eggplant, and peppers. While these may be fine for most people, they are all big no-no's for people with skin conditions.[85]

For the first time in her life, Kim had relief. She now understood how to heal her skin, in a natural food-related way. At thirty-five with a healthy Max at her side, Kim began a new chapter. She started by cleaning out all her kitchen cupboards, the pantry, the refrigerator, etc. She threw away every single unhealthy food item. She also called her close friends and family and told them, many for the first time, what she was doing. She told them she needed their support to help change her diet and her life.

Kim changed everything. She even went completely vegan. This was not necessary for her skin; it was a choice she made. She was on a mission to heal herself. In the beginning, this complete change was easy because Kim was so incredibly motivated. It was also easier in the beginning because she saw results almost immediately. Seeing spots fade away kept her motivation high. And though she missed things like mimosas

---

85 "What Are Nightshade Vegetables? – Dr. Axe." 2017. *Dr. Axe.* https://draxe.com/night-shade-vegetables (accessed April 28, 2017).

when she was out to brunch—because of course, brunch in the city means mimosas—she was determined to see all her spots gone.

For one entire year, Kim was a strict vegan. She ate nothing but whole grains, vegetables and fruits, nuts and seeds, and legumes and beans. That was it. This may seem like a limited variety, but Kim became obsessed with cooking and she concocted some wonderful meals. She became creative in the kitchen and tried new recipes. Kim missed carbs and sweets, so she found new ways to make cookies—vegan cookies with almond flour, raisins, and pure maple syrup. It's difficult to not go out to eat when you're living in Manhattan, but for that first year, Kim asked all her friends if they could go to vegan or vegetarian restaurants, or restaurants where she could get a ton of vegetables or a big salad. She was determined.

Month ten into this one-year excursion, Kim's skin was 100% completely clear. For the first time in almost twenty years she had clear skin. She described this as "freeing as all hell." She had been in what she called psoriasis prison. Now she was free. Kim was literally in tears when she described this feeling to me. One day soon after this ten-month period, she went to work in a tee shirt. For the first time in decades she didn't have to hide her elbows. She was so proud of her arms and wanted to show them off. At the same time, she said she was in the bathroom every hour looking at her elbows to make sure they were still okay. She was so scared it was going to come back. She was so scared because that's all she knew. She had lived with psoriasis for so long that hiding her skin was a natural thing for Kim. She didn't know what it was like to not live with it.

This new freedom was amazing. Amazing! Kim felt "normal" again. She had been so disgusted by it her whole life. Imagine being disgusted by your own skin? No longer. Now she felt human again. It was a surreal moment. She had healed her skin and kept thinking, *I don't have to go to a dermatologist ever again!* Kim was the one in control now—of her skin, of her health, of her life.

Kim also realized that her body was communicating with her. Her body was talking and Kim learned how to listen. Her body needed nutrients. It needed nourishment and Kim hadn't been listening. For her entire life she wasn't listening. Now Kim listens to her body. This is crucial. We all need to do this! Your body is talking to you. Try meeting it halfway by acting on the messages you hear.

For about a year and a half to two years Kim had clear skin. She was healed. During this time, she met her husband Mike. It wasn't obvious from the outside that she had ever had a problem with her skin as it was now perfectly clear, so he would never have known just by looking at her, but Kim shared her story with him. It was fairly obvious in other ways that this was a big part of her life. She was blogging about her journey and she was still mostly vegetarian, though she did incorporate some wild-caught salmon at times and once in a while some organic chicken.

During the first few weeks of dating Mike, her diet had started to shift. We all know what happens when you fall in love. You lose focus on *you* and become part of *we*. They were going out to dinner a lot, and Kim would sometimes splurge and share dessert with him. She also found herself drinking more. From listening to her body, Kim knew she had to monitor her alcohol intake. She could handle a little, but she found herself having wine with dinner whenever they went out to eat. Kim was in a conundrum of sorts. She knew she had to watch her diet more carefully and get back on track, but she was also in la-la land and in love. Kim admitted that she felt a little invincible. Her psoriasis was gone, so there was a little of that "It's gone. I'm healed. I'm done. It's all good." factor going on.

Three months into her relationship with Mike, Kim had a horrible accident, and she was in recovery after a major surgery for about a year. Her regimented diet went out the window. She was off the alkaline wagon completely. She had to rely on hospital food, people cooking for her, and people ordering out for her. She had very little choice in what she was eating. When people are already going out of their way to help feed you, it's difficult to ask them to make you an organic green smoothie instead of that grilled cheese sandwich. It's also difficult to care when you are that out of sorts and in pain.

Not to mention depressed. Kim was stuck in bed for months. Anyone would be depressed. She couldn't enjoy life with Mike the way she wanted; she couldn't do any of the things she loved; she couldn't work; she was on a lot of medication. Kim could barely go to the bathroom by herself. It was such a depressing time that Kim didn't care about the kinds of food she was putting into her body. So the combination of medication, depression, and eating crap resulted in her psoriasis returning in a very short amount of time.

This was a huge blow to Kim. If she wasn't already depressed about her accident, surgery, and long recovery, her psoriasis put the last nail in the coffin. She was so disappointed in herself. She had let her guard down and allowed the psoriasis to come back. Kim knew what she had to do to keep it away, and while that knowledge was some comfort, she was spiraling down into a deeper depression. It was a struggle—every day. She had months of physical therapy and finally went back to work, with crutches, but struggled through each day.

Then the day came when Mike fully understood what her psoriasis was all about. She hadn't been hiding it from him. He knew about it, but had never seen it because when they met her skin was totally clear. She'd never had it since she met him, and in some ways she didn't even realize it was back in full force. Maybe she didn't want to let herself acknowledge it. She remembers they were watching television, and Mike put his arm around her and his hand fell just to the right spot on her elbow. He felt that rough, dry skin of psoriasis. He said, "Oh, is this psoriasis? Is this what it is?" He had never seen it before. Kim was mortified. But she knew this was the guy she wanted to marry, and the psoriasis wasn't going anywhere any time soon. It was a bad moment for Kim. Her ego was beating her up. She never wanted Mike to see it or feel it and now here it was: full-blown psoriasis. Again.

This opened up the conversation and she was able to tell him that she needed to get back on track. She told him that she needed to get back to her strict vegan alkaline way of eating. "It's time. I have to do this." Mike was completely there for her. He said, "Okay, you have my support; just tell me what you need." So, this time together with Mike, they emptied out their kitchen and Kim got back on track. This time was slightly different, though, as she was no longer living in the city with a farmers' market across the street where she could get all her vegetables. They were living out on Long Island, where you have to drive to get anywhere. Before she only had to worry about her and Max, so if she wanted broccoli for dinner, it was no big deal. Now she had to feed Mike as well. Meals required more thought and had to be planned out ahead of time. It was an entirely new lifestyle Kim had to get used to.

A few months later, Kim found herself extremely frustrated because the diet wasn't working. She was doing everything she had done before, but not getting the same results. Her skin wasn't healing and she couldn't understand why. One night she was pacing back and forth saying, "I just don't understand why. Why isn't it working? I'm doing exactly what I did before. What am I missing? There's something I'm missing here." Then Mike said, "You know you're under a lot of stress at work, right? Do you think that might have something to do with it?" Lightbulb!

Well, of course it does, Kim thought. Her job was putting an inordinate amount of stress on her body. So much so that some nights she would be in tears. Bingo. Kim's body was trying to tell her something, and this time Mike heard it loud and clear. Her body was telling her to decrease the stress and either quit the job or figure something out. Somehow she needed to decrease stress. This new piece of knowledge led Kim to practice more self-care and self-love. She started making a point of caring for Kim. She started getting monthly massages, listening to music on the way home instead of working, going for walks without her phone, meditation, and other things that helped her relax. These things weren't helping her skin heal necessarily, but Kim knew they were important in helping her unwind and focus on self.

Kim started practicing self-care and learning more and more how to love herself. She was learning how to talk to herself in a nicer, more loving way. This was a big breakthrough. Instead of the negative self-talk a lot of us have in our heads, Kim's self-talk was becoming more positive and loving. She was learning to love her skin whether or not it had bumps on it. She understood that she needed to love it and stop hating it. This was not easy. Kim called it a constant emotional roller coaster. But she knew it was necessary for her healing. Not just for her skin, but for Kim the person.

She noticed a shift when she started talking to her skin and saying loving things to it. Kim began a ritual in her morning shower where she would thank her body for working so hard for her. She started to love on herself and stopped hating herself.

For people with skin issues, it's on the outside for everyone to see. You already feel terrible about it. Most people with skin issues hate their skin. They ask, why me? They look at it all the time. They're disgusted by it. It makes them feel ugly and self-conscious—in everything they do, everywhere they go. It destroys their self-esteem. So this was a huge shift for Kim to stop the hate and turn on the love. It became a daily habit for

Kim to start her day with love and end her day with love—for her skin, for her body, for herself.

This shift in how Kim felt about herself started to heal her skin as well. It reinforced for her that nutrition is not just about food. Who and what you surround yourself with, how you talk to yourself and others, your spiritual practice, your physical activity, your relationships, and self-love are all part of the equation.

The formula that finally healed Kim's skin is: self-love; making her happiness a priority; having healthy relationships with people, food, money, and her body; and being able to alleviate stress. These are the things that are most important to Kim. These are the things she works on a little bit every day. These days if Kim gets a random spot on her leg, she gives it love and practices more self-care. She knows what she needs and then she gives it to herself.

Kim's journey led her to the knowledge that she wanted to help others with skin conditions. She knows there are millions of people in the world struggling every day with the same anxiety she did. She knows she has a gift to share. She didn't know how to go about this, though. She wasn't sure how to make a living at this and make money doing it. Then the Institute for Integrative Nutrition fell into her lap, because that's how the universe works. Today Kim is a Certified International Health Coach and is passionate about helping others heal their skin.

A couple of months before I interviewed Kim, she had her first book, *Ps– It's All About Love: How a Painful Journey with Psoriasis Became a Life Devoted to Healing Others*, published—a much more in-depth look at her journey to healing her skin. "Ps" is short for psoriasis. She knows it will help thousands if not millions of people. She said that's why it was born. That's why it was written.

Inspiration:

When I asked Kim if there was anything positive and/or inspirational that made her suffering worth it, she responded by saying she is very grateful that she had psoriasis. She knows that others with psoriasis may cringe when they read this, but for Kim, if she'd never had psoriasis, she wouldn't be able to help people with their skin issues. She can't help but feel that her journey of learning about nutrition and self-love paved the way for her to work her life's mission. She knows that anyone can use these tools and live this lifestyle and heal him- or herself from the inside out. All of us have the power to take control of our health and heal ourselves. Of course, doctors are needed. But for issues like this, we can heal ourselves with nutrition and self-love. Kim is living proof.

Advice:

I also asked Kim what advice she can give to people in their darkest moments, and what pulled her through? She said when she thinks of the darkest moment, she goes back to when she was sitting on her toilet, hysterically crying, screaming to the universe, why me? She was in so much emotional pain. But she knows people in worse shape. She knows a man with genital psoriasis that is so raw and cracked he bleeds. It's incredibly painful. He can't date and has tried to end his life a few times because of it. This is the advice Kim gave to him.

"Your body is talking to you and you haven't been listening to it. Now it's time to listen. You're in the most helpless spot you could ever be in. Now is the time to make a choice. You either believe that you can heal or you allow it to control you. That's the choice. You allow it to control you and keep you paralyzed and in a dark place—or you choose to control it."

Everything in life is a choice. We can choose to listen to our bodies and take control of our health. You make a choice that you are not going to live with this pain anymore. Once you make that decision, something lifts in us. It's like you have some control back. Then you can begin the healing process ... one baby step at a time. For the man above, his first step was to talk with Kim. Isn't it time we all start to listen to our bodies and find people we can actually talk to?

Contact:

Kim is an International Certified Health Coach, published author, speaker, and all-around amazing person. She is passionate about helping others heal their skin conditions. If you have skin issues and want to take that first step, contact Kim today through her website: http://www.healingmyskin.com/

Chapter 14

Becky: Lupus

Functional medicine practitioners treat your body's ecosystem. We get rid of the bad stuff, put in the good stuff and because your body is an intelligent system—it does the rest.

—Mark Hyman, MD

Becky

Growing up, Becky was frequently sick. She was one of those kids who had a cold and then immediately after got bronchitis. As she got older, it got continually worse. It was really bad after she had her first child at the age of twenty. Soon after, she got married at the age of twenty-three and was at the doctor's office every two weeks. There was always something new, either a new infection or a new cold, from ears-nose-throat to kidneys; every system was affected during the months shortly after she was married.

By almost twenty-four, Becky was pretty much in bed. She barely left her bedroom. She would get sick repeatedly with some kind of infection, which was, as you would expect, treated with antibiotics. Her symptoms were all over the place. She couldn't sleep, then she was sleeping too much; she also had intermittent fevers. Can you say "miserable"?

Fed up, Becky finally went to her primary care physician, who essentially told her she was very young to be having all these issues and sent her to see a rheumatologist. Rheumatology is a medical specialty for people with "the more than 100 types of arthritis along with the complex diseases, including lupus, systemic sclerosis (scleroderma), vasculitis and inflammatory muscle disease."[86]

Of course Becky went; and she had a horrible experience. She said the rheumatologist was awful. She was a little Russian woman who came into the examining room and started grabbing Becky. She was assessing her and checking all her joints and yelling at Becky, saying, "Don't you realize these are all swollen?" To Becky, though, this was normal, so why would she think they were swollen?

This little Russian doctor was incredibly rude to Becky. She was mean and scared the you-know-what out of her, and Becky left her office in tears. As Becky was leaving, the doctor handed her some pamphlets and said, "Well you have one of these two things." One of the pamphlets was for rheumatoid arthritis (RA), the other for lupus.

---

86   2017. https://weillcornell.org/rheumatology (accessed February 14, 2017).

Becky went home, and having no knowledge of her own at that point, started researching online. If you've ever searched online for rheumatoid arthritis (RA), images will display of horribly disfigured hands and fingers. I was squirming in my seat looking at them. Imagine Becky—at 24—looking at these images?

Fortunately (or unfortunately, depending on how you look at it), Becky did not have rheumatoid arthritis. She did, however, have lupus. Becky thought, okay, I guess that's better than the other one; I don't know. So she went back to the doctor, the little Russian one, who was in her face saying that Becky needed IV treatment that very day. She needed IV immunosuppressant drugs, like immediately. Becky looked at her and said, "No."

The doctor hadn't explained anything to her; she said nothing about prognosis; she didn't explain what lupus was, how it progresses or how it would impact Becky's life. She didn't tell Becky anything she needed to hear. Becky needed to hear options; how long; what would her prognosis be if she did the treatment? The doctor gave her nothing. So Becky left.

Then she cried. And, then she found a new doctor. Fortunately, Becky has a friend who is a drug representative for arthritic medication who told her, "Do not ever go there again. Here is a new doctor."

The new doctor was wonderful! She had a beautiful bedside manner—a complete 180-degree turnaround from the little mean Russian doctor. She looked at Becky's lab work and confirmed the diagnosis. She said the other doctor was right, though her treatment approach was wrong. No kidding! She started Becky on a high dose of Plaquenil,[87] which is known as an anti-malarial medication, but it's used for autoimmune diseases such as rheumatoid arthritis and lupus as well.

Unfortunately, the side effects of the medication were worse than what Becky had been experiencing from the lupus. She started losing hair; she became an insomniac; she began to overeat; she couldn't drive from dizziness; she started having all these awful issues. Becky was so dizzy from the medication that she couldn't even stand up and walk down the hallway. This lasted for weeks.

She remembers calling the doctor and telling her that she felt like hell, that she couldn't function, that this was worse than what it was before. The doctor told her, "It takes time to adjust, but I think your dosage is too high." Apparently, they had put her on the highest dose to try and knock it out quickly. Since that didn't work they lowered it, and within six months, Becky was a normal functioning person.

Lupus, or systemic lupus erythematosus (SLE), is an autoimmune disease, which we've learned is where the body attacks itself; it essentially "produces antibodies against healthy cells and tissues." The difference in lupus versus other autoimmune diseases is that in lupus, the antibodies attack part of the cells' nucleus. For those of us who are not scientists, the nucleus is where most of our body's genetic material is stored and it pretty much is the core operating point, telling our body

---

87 "Plaquenil Uses, Dosage & Side Effects – Drugs.Com." 2017. *Drugs.Com.* https://www. drugs.com/plaquenil.html (accessed March 6, 2017).

what to do and how to act to survive. For my geek friends, think of this as the central processing unit (CPU). The CPU handles all the various instructions it receives from the hardware and software on the computer; it processes instructions. Another analogy could be like an air traffic controller, directing all the different airplanes in the vicinity where and when to turn, when to land and take off, etc. The nucleus acts in a similar fashion; it receives information and coordinates activity, directing other parts to do their thing ... The bottom line is if the nucleus is confused, imagine all the negative results it can have on your body. Common symptoms of lupus are joint pain, fever, and fatigue, which Becky had in spades. The causes or triggers of lupus are still being researched, though doctors feel that it's a "combination of genetic, environmental and hormonal factors."[88]

Becky stayed on the Plaquenil for years and had many of the issues that come with autoimmune disorders, such as polycystic ovary syndrome (PCOS). During this time, Becky got pregnant, which her doctors told her couldn't happen. She was also in the middle of an incredibly stressful nursing school program. So, she got pregnant during the most stressful time of her life, when they told her she couldn't. Well, of course, this put her immediately into the high-risk category, which meant Becky and her baby had to be monitored on a weekly basis.

Becky was miserable. The testing seemed to be nonstop. She had insomnia the entire time, which worsened all of the

---

88 Wellness, Health, Mind & Spirit Body, and Autoimmune Disorders. 2017. "Lupus – Dr. Weil's Condition Care Guide." *Drweil.Com.* https://www.drweil.com/health-wellness/body-mind-spirit/autoimmune-disorders/lupus/ (accessed February 15, 2017).

lupus symptoms that had previously improved. Plus, she was constantly sick. Becky ended up dropping out of nursing school. She just couldn't commit to the pressure and stress, and she certainly couldn't keep throwing up during her clinical rounds. She finished out the semester and told them she would be back.

After delivering her daughter, a healthy eight-pound spitfire named Mia, Becky decided that she needed to re-center her life. Her oldest was seven at the time, in school, and Becky wanted to be at home with her little one. So she took some time to figure it all out.

Her doctors had told her to continue her medications throughout her pregnancy and even after. Becky, for some reason, didn't like this and decided to discontinue the meds. She was breastfeeding and was concerned about the medication being transferred into her tiny daughter. She had also been concerned while she was pregnant, but knew the risk of not taking the meds was higher than harming her baby.

Against her doctor's wishes, Becky stopped taking the Plaquenil. Her youngest just turned four and she hasn't been on any medication since shortly after her birth. Throughout this time a lot of things happened. First of all, being pregnant does crazy things to your hormones—sometimes good and sometimes bad. Knowing what she knows now about autoimmune issues, Becky realized that the hormone shift from her first pregnancy triggered everything else. This is when everything started going downhill. She started getting rashes on her face among other things, and her doctors wrote it off as hormones.

Now she understands that there was an underlying issue that was never addressed. After having Mia, her little one, she discontinued the meds and decided to go back to work to figure out what she truly wanted in life. Thinking back to when she was in nursing school, Becky realized that she didn't want to push medications as a nurse after having a change in perspective around pharmaceuticals and after stopping her own prescribed meds. That path was no longer an option.

When she was able, Becky went back to work in a local pain management office. She told me she had never worked in pain management before—and never will again. The good thing, though, was that in this office, she met a functional medical practitioner. After a conversation in the lunchroom about her health journey, this woman said, "I want you. I want to teach you everything."

Becky had no idea who she was and wondered, who are you and what are you going to teach me? And yet, that moment right there changed Becky's life. This doctor brought Becky into the functional medicine fold and helped Becky heal herself. According to Dr. Mark Hyman, functional medicine looks at the whole system that is the human body. It's a holistic approach that "seeks to identify and address the root causes of disease, and views the body as one integrated system, not a collection of independent organs divided up by medical specialties."[89]

---

89 Articles, Latest, Ask FAQs, Mark's Minutes, TV Media, and MD Mark Hyman. 2017. "About Functional Medicine – Dr. Mark Hyman." *Dr. Mark Hyman.* http://drhyman.com/about-2/about-functional-medicine/ (accessed February 15, 2017).

With this doctor, Becky learned about gut health, which was the turning point in her healing journey. The combination of whole foods and balancing her gut bacteria was the key to Becky's healing. These things sound so simple, but many people overlook them and end up sick. Becky started working with this doctor and learned everything she possibly could. During her tenure there, she ran an opioid dependency program, diets groups, and did just about everything she could learn and do.

While there, she heard about the Institute for Integrative Nutrition, in which she almost immediately enrolled. Becky decided to leave that job and take a year off so that she could focus on school and be at home with her kids.

During this journey to health, Becky found her triggers. For example, she knows she can't have sugar. This is something she focuses on with her clients. Everyone has triggers for whatever ailment they suffer from, and it's important to identify these triggers and learn how to avoid them. Whether it's arthritis or irritable bowel syndrome (IBS) or Crohn's— it's not always textbook. In other words, there is not always a cookie-cutter answer. It's not always "if x then y." As bio-individual unique humans, our bodies are as different as grains of sand on a beach. Thus two people with the same health issues may have entirely different triggers.

Before Becky realized she had any health issues, she, like many others, ate the Standard American Diet (SAD). The SAD is typically high in animal fats, bad fats, and processed foods, and low in fiber and plant-based foods. Growing up on a farm meant typical meals consisted of meat and potatoes. And by meat, she meant red meat. Becky now knows red meat is no friend of hers.[90]

Her diet today consists of the most natural form of any food. For example, she avoids sugar, though she may have raw honey periodically. Becky also stays away from breads and pastas; anything that breaks down into sugars. Thus even fruit is extremely limited. She focuses on complex carbohydrates such as brown rice and quinoa, lots of vegetables, and chicken.

She tried to go vegetarian at one point, but found she couldn't do it. She didn't like it. So Becky does eat meat, specifically chicken, two to three times per week. Once she added poultry back into her diet, she realized she actually likes it. So as she puts it, "she's not religiously vegetarian." Becky loves to cook and says that cooking with meat, chicken, etc., is irreplaceable. She feels it may be a comfort thing.

Today, Becky is a health coach practitioner and she absolutely loves it. She is healthy and still on no medications. She says her healing was a lot about her being angry. She was fed up with the ways of modern medicine. She didn't know where to start until she met the functional medicine doctor, who happened to be vegetarian. At first Becky said, "I don't know how you can do that," but then working with this doctor, she was required to teach about it. They say that the best way to learn something is to teach it. Well, Becky figured another

---

90   2017.   http://www.askdrsears.com/topics/feeding-eating/family-nutrition/standard-american-diet-sad (accessed February 9, 2017).

way to learn about it was to do it. The first thing she cut out was milk, and she realized she felt really good. Prior to this, she used to eat yogurt every day in the morning, not realizing it made her feel awful. So basically, Becky says: you don't know until you try.

The funny thing is, most people don't want to try. But when they hear stories like Becky's—they may try something different. Becky is very grateful that she figured all this out at a relatively early age. Had she waited even another ten years, imagine how damaged her internal systems would be? It would have been so much more difficult to get back on track— if she could have. By that point the damage to her body might have been irreparable. She is very grateful that it came into her life at the right time.

Inspiration:

Becky believes that her life up to this point has been all about the journey and not about the destination. Throughout her suffering with an autoimmune disease and her journey to get well, Becky became a stronger and more powerful version of herself. She became the woman who was able to pull herself up emotionally and physically, instead of relying on others to do so. Becky became truly independent, but she also found strength in actually asking for help and in helping others.

Advice:

It was difficult for Becky to put the emotional strength she developed into words, but she offered this:

"The best advice I could ever give someone in their deepest darkest moments would be to find an anchor and hold on, because this too shall pass. The ability to anchor your mind, body and spirit to a place of healing and peace is so important to those suffering and in a dark place. Finding your anchor is key to becoming stable emotionally and physically. My anchor was/is my husband and my children."

Contact:

If you've been inspired by Becky's story or simply want to get in touch with her, reach out via email at: wellnessrxbybecky@gmail.com, or find her on Facebook @beckymartinhealthcoach

PART FIVE

Body Or Mind?
When Food
Becomes Your
Enemy And Not
Your Medicine

Chapter 15

Depression, Weight Disorders, or Simply Your Body Lacking the Nutrients It Needs?

Health is a state of complete physical, mental, and social wellbeing, and not merely the absence of disease or infirmity.

World Health Organization, 1948

I am starting this chapter with a quote from the World Health Organization (WHO). While I may not agree with many, many things that happen in that organization—another book—I can say that they do an excellent job with statistics. Therefore, when I refer to WHO it is mostly for their data accrual and dissemination of information. Funny, though: I completely agree with the above quote that health is a state of well-being and not an absence of illness!

It is astonishing to hear that Americans suffer from one of the highest levels of mental illness—more than any other country in the world. How can that be, you might ask, considering we live in one of the wealthiest nations in the world? How can that be when we have education, psychologists, counselors, and treatment specialists, and all sorts of helping programs—some free and some paid for by insurance or the government?

How is it that we are blessed enough to live in a world where we have progressed so far as to not hold such a stigma against mental illness, that we can encourage treatment, not have to hide away, and yet, our numbers and stats just keep growing and growing? And, that is not a good thing.

An article popped up on April 17, 2017 that caught my eye written by Dr. Mercola (a traditional doctor who has moved into completely holistic realms) that stated:

According to the World Health Organization (WHO), depression is now the leading cause of ill health and disability worldwide, affecting an estimated 322 million people worldwide, including more than 16 million Americans. Globally, rates of depression increased by 18 percent between 2005 and 2015.

According to the U.S. National Institute of Mental Health, 11 percent of Americans over the age of 12 are on antidepressant drugs. Among women in their 40 and 50s, 1 in 4 is on antidepressants.

Depression is also strongly linked to an increased risk for substance abuse, diseases such as diabetes and heart disease, and suicide.[91]

91 2017. http://articles.mercola.com/sites/articles/archive/2017/04/13/depression-leading-cause-of-illness-disability-worldwide (accessed April 17, 2017).

This particular article went on to discuss that these statistics are low, and in the United States 50% of the population is underdiagnosed and undertreated, and in third world countries it is closer to 80%.[92] These numbers take my breath away. It is agonizing to think that this many people are suffering in the world and that we are not getting to the reason why.

Let me share with you that I am not talking about the healthy depression that sets in after major life changes or events, the one that is a natural and necessary part of life. What I am talking about is that deeper level of depression that moves into "clinical" territory.

According to WHO, America is the third most depressed country after India and China. You read this correctly! The third—why is that? What do we seriously have to be depressed about?

The DSM-5, the *Diagnostic and Statistical Manual of Mental Disorders*, Fifth Edition, that psychiatrists use to define the level of mental pathology is more than 500 pages long, and each page is jam-packed with various forms of mental illness. How can we as a world be suffering with so much bipolar depression, anxiety disorders, mood disorders, psychotic episodes, developmental disorders, and then so much autism, Attention Deficit Disorder (ADD), Attention Deficit Hyperactivity Disorder (ADHD), drug abuse, eating disorders, sleeping disorders, and the list goes on?

Since there are books and books and materials and materials written about this topic, I am not going to focus on

---

92   Ibid.

"treating" mental disorders. I'll leave that to the professionals. However, I do want to address a few important facts, from the perspective of a layperson, which I think would be valuable for anyone out there suffering from feelings of blame, depression, guilt, anxiety, dread, and low self-worth, etc.

The first is to look at your life and determine what significant stressors are going on—because if you score high on life-changing events that are all transpiring at one time, like a death, a move, a divorce, a lost relationship, lost health, a lost pet ... all in a short period, you *should* be depressed! You should feel anxious and worried and overwhelmed. That *is* a natural and healthy response. This means you need to give yourself some attention and self-care and a break. You need to allow yourself time to heal. If you need some medication to get you through, so be it. Sometimes life is hard, really hard, but if there is a way you can give yourself time and remain as holistic as possible, such as with Bach herbal remedies, Kava Kava, Valerian tea, St. John's Wort (careful not to mix if you are already on an antidepressant) and not skip right to the Prozacs, Wellbutrins, while topping them off with Xanax and a sleeping pill, you may find your healing comes more quickly. Every prescription medication has its own side effects, whereas with herbs there are none. You need to carefully do your research and find a knowledgeable coach, but you can learn what your body likes and what can help heal you the fastest.

In order to determine how depressed you are, a psychologist friend of mine shared that she likes to recommend people do a self-test that takes about 20 minutes and that garners quick but pretty accurate results. Before you stop reading, run to the computer, and take the test, make sure you are not missing one very important piece: if you score within 40–80% and already suffer from a chronic or serious physical illness, this will influence the results and you will understandably be suffering from some depression. This will make more sense after you take the test.

Now, go ahead and complete the test at https://www.psychologytoday.com/test/3889 to learn how you are doing with depression and if you should explore getting a little extra help.

The second most valuable piece of information she shared is that if you do this test and you have only minimal physical problems and you show up as clinically depressed, then this tells you that you need to take some form of action, psychologically. It means clinically your serotonin is not firing and therefore it needs a boost. Think of it like this—you are either pregnant or you're not. It's the same thing with neurotransmitters like serotonin, norepinephrine, dopamine, etc.: they are either firing or not. If your neurotransmitters are not firing, then something has gone wrong and they need support either with serotonin reuptake inhibitors or some other compound to physically get them to fire again. A drained pool of neurotransmitters can very rarely make it back to full operation without a boost. Time and natural healing will do it for some, but you are at a critical enough point that you need to seek some form of help. Your body needs a boost to pull you out of the depression, and a great therapist or coach will help you succeed so much faster.

Another important point from the psychologist was to make sure that *before* you ever let a psychologist, psychiatrist, doctor, or counselor make a diagnosis of any mental disorder, you must first rule out any type of physical disorder. As a trained Ivy League clinical psychologist, unlike most who have come through the traditional higher education programs, she found that over 70 percent of the "depressed" population she saw had been misdiagnosed. This is alarming. One of the most major illnesses, again misdiagnosed, can be a thyroid disorder, and if the gland is hyperactive you can be prone to anxiety. If it is underactive you can feel so sluggish you just can't get moving, and in time that weighs on you; you think you are less valuable than you are and you, of course, become depressed. She also recommends that before you treat for depression you check for adrenal fatigue, sleep disorders, autoimmune illnesses, and the list goes on. Needless to say, if you already have a chronic illness or terminal illness, you are going to have down and blue days. Horrifying to think, but some of her terminal patients were told they were depressed and needed antidepressants on top of all the other medications, which did not help in most cases.

I am sharing this so that if there is only one piece of advice you take from the people I interviewed, make sure you are technically "clinically' depressed and that you are not suffering from something else. On a physical level, believe it or not, a serious candida or yeast infection can cause so much havoc in your body you will present to an unknowing psychologist as bipolar—now who ever shares that information? *If* you are in the midst of toxic overload, you could be struggling with manic or psychotic breaks—who tells you that? Again, if you have a history, yes, a genetic predisposition, then it is likely this psychiatric diagnosis is accurate, but there are so many ways to strengthen your body so that you don't live with depression or mania or attacks that it is worth researching more—becoming your own investigator. If you are a child or living in a house with a psychotic parent and it turns out that there is an over-growth of mold or lead paint in the house, not one of you may have a psychiatric disorder at all. You are toxic and once that is cleaned up, the mental illness will go away! Imagine that. (Again, do not take this as medical advice; seek out a profes-sional, but being armed with information and finding a thera-pist or professional who honors that versus scoffs at it means that you are going to get the help you need.)

The other area of disorders that fall under mental disor-ders are those related to weight. So many people struggle with food issues and body distortion because of the advertisements on TV and what we are taught is normal by watching tiny-framed actors and actresses and comparing ourselves, but the truth is that we come in all different sizes and dimensions. The other truth is that if our body has the nutrients and care it needs, it will automatically move to the perfect weight for us. That might mean losing weight, but it might also mean gaining weight. When you are on a weight yo-yo, it is a sign that you have some form of nutrient issues you need to ad-dress, and yes, best to address the psychological factors that are feeding into the distress and bad habits.

Again, referring to the DSM-5, the *Diagnostic and Statistical Manual of Mental Disorders*, Fifth Edition, there are the traditional clinical eating disorders that now most peo-ple have heard something about. These include: anorexia ner-vosa, where people practically starve themselves to death and still feel they are fat; bulimia, where people force themselves to throw up so as to not gain weight from calories; binge eating, where they can't stop eating and overindulge but then the following days restrict their calories in hopes they won't gain weight; and/or a combination of them. However, there is also a more recent recognition of another disorder that is not officially in the DSM-5, and that is called orthorexia. Orthorexia "was coined in 1998 and means an obsession with proper or 'healthful' eating. Although being aware of and concerned with the nutritional quality of the food you eat isn't a problem in and of itself, people with orthorexia become so fixated on so-called 'healthy eating' that they actually damage their own well-being."[93] This is where the individual is so obsessed with the exact calorie count that they often won't go out to social places for fear they will not know or will mess up their calorie count for the day.

One of our women shares that so many times in our society, people are judged by appearances. By how they look, the car they drive, the house they own, the clothes they wear, their speech patterns, etc. Yet, often, the most seemingly fit and healthy among us are the ones who need the most help. They are the ones with low self-esteem, guilt, judgment, and insecurity issues. This is something the health, diet, and fitness industry all play on for profit, and the movie and advertising industry plays on to sell products. It is really important to address both the psychological and physical reasons behind eating disorders, but the good news is sometimes just recognizing and putting a name to the disorder can put it in

---

93   "Orthorexia." 2017. *National Eating Disorders Association.* https://www.nationale-atingdisorders.org/learn/by-eating-disorder/other/orthorexia (accessed May 8, 2017).

perspective and get you to start to heal. Remember, your body wants and craves the proper nutrients and care to thrive.

Now that I have shared the above important information, I would like to share the personal stories that deal with general health, weight issues, energy questions at times, depression, and the will to live, which may mean nothing more than a lack of good nutrients, healthy bacteria, and reinforcing minerals to support your genes ... it may feel like you don't have the energy to move or function because you truly just physically do not. Your mind may be ready but your weak body just can't comply.

My advice, before you call yourself crazy: do a little self-test, or reach out to some other women who have been there. You may just find you will be calling the diagnosticians crazy and learn that you were never mentally challenged at all!

Chapter 16

Lauren: Binging, Working Out, and Orthorexia

I have come to believe that caring for myself is not self-indulgent. Caring for myself is an act of survival.

—*Audre Lorde*

Lauren

Lauren's story started when she was very young. She doesn't remember an exact age, but sometime in elementary school Lauren noticed she was getting comments about her weight from some of the other kids. What made this even worse was that she got picked on by her siblings in the safety of her own home.

As she got a little older, she would overhear comments from boys saying things like they would go out with her if she lost some weight. They even made fun of her for being tall and having freckles. It was a difficult childhood for Lauren, and from a very young age, she became self-conscious about her body.

At around the age of eleven, Lauren began to eat uncontrollably to cope with her feelings. She remembers not having many friends, while her brother and sister were very popular. Her siblings would often be out of the house doing things with their friends and never wanted to include her, so Lauren would sit at home. Alone. She would plop herself down on the couch and go from the refrigerator to the television to the cupboard, grabbing one thing after another. This bingeing had the effect of numbing her feelings with food until she literally made herself sick.

Once her siblings came home with their friends in tow, they would tease her and say things like her only exercise was going to the fridge and opening it and that she should just kill herself. Kids can be so cruel. There were a lot of comments like that and a lot of days like that. All of this took its toll and Lauren became a very angry and depressed kid. She almost felt like she was lazy, never wanting to get up off the couch. But the truth was, she was stuck in a cycle of feeling like crap and not knowing what to do.

For a long time, Lauren was suicidal. She would continually think about wanting to die. She hated herself that much— to the point that every night she was thinking about wanting to die. Yet, there was always this tiny voice in the back of her head telling her to hang in there, that she was going to be fine, to just push through.

Lauren was fourteen before she got fed up. She was sick and tired of being angry. She was done with lashing out at others and then hating herself. Somehow she thought that losing weight was the solution. Lauren felt that if she lost weight, it would be a turning point in her life and people would finally accept her. So, she told her mom that she wanted to lose fifty pounds. Lauren's mom made a deal with her—if she made it to the halfway point, her mom would buy her a gym membership.

This time, Lauren was serious and she put herself on a diet. Her first diet. At fourteen.

How many of us have been there?

Lauren started working out to exercise videos in her home three times per week and within a few months had released 33 pounds. True to her word, Lauren's mom got her that gym membership, and she experienced that first weight loss high. For the first time in her life, Lauren was hearing comments about how good she looked. All of a sudden, she was being accepted. Boys were starting to pay attention to her and she was making new friends.

This experience led her to the false and dangerous belief that her weight determined her worth.

Lauren kept that weight off for a long time.

When she was 19, Lauren went into the military and was stationed in England. She started eating a lot of the local food and drinking a lot of alcohol, and as a result gained weight again. During this entire time, Lauren continued with the binge eating behavior that even followed her to the United Kingdom.

At the time, though, she had no idea she had Binge Eating Disorder (BED) or that there even was such a thing as Binge Eating Disorder. As a kid she had learned about anorexia and bulimia, but back then BED wasn't well-known. Lauren knew she wasn't anorexic or bulimic, but she felt out of control. At times her eating was so out of control that she felt there was something seriously wrong with her. When you can't put a name to it—it makes you depressed and angry.

So even though no one was making any comments about her weight gain, Lauren was hard on herself and went back into her previous diet-binge cycle. She was able to lose some weight and keep it off and she got back into the groove, so to speak.

Then Lauren got into a relationship. We all know what typically happens when you fall in love and begin that nesting stage—you let your guard down, you let someone else in, you focus on that other person and less on yourself, and you gain weight. Lauren got so comfortable, and was having a great time, that she gained all her weight back again. She stopped taking care of herself. She thought that her boyfriend loved her and that she didn't have to focus so much on her diet and exercise anymore. She forgot about self-love.

Lauren stopped going to the gym as much, and somehow she thought she could eat the same foods in the same amounts that her boyfriend could—which was a lot. But we all know men's bodies are very different than women's bodies. We have different metabolisms and we have different bone and muscle structures. Without thinking about it, the weight crept back on.

One night, about six months into the relationship, Lauren got this intuitive feeling that her boyfriend wasn't as attracted to her as he had been in the beginning. So, bravely, she asked him if he had lost some of his attraction for her since she had gained weight. He replied honestly and said yes. Lauren was devastated and began that familiar spiral of crying and wanting to die and hating herself. She could not understand why she couldn't just get herself under control. She felt that she would be struggling with her weight and her body for her entire life. That this struggle would always continue.

So, again, Lauren went into the diet cycle. This time was slightly different, though, as she got into strength training and decided she wanted to compete on stage in bikini competitions. At this point Lauren had separated from the military and began a body transformation challenge. She remained with Jason, her boyfriend, although now it was long distance, which gave her a little more freedom to focus on herself. So she did a transformation challenge and got great results. For the next two years she focused on bodybuilding. Lauren was on cloud nine! She thought she had found her answer and her community.

But, the reality was that every single day Lauren was beating herself up. She was checking her body out in the mirror, she was pinching herself, she was measuring her fat, and she was fixating on her caloric intake and her macros (i.e., grams of protein, carbohydrates, and fat). This became an obsession. She was so preoccupied with these things that she decided to go to school to become a registered dietician. She thought this would finally give her all the answers. This was going to fix whatever was wrong with her. She was going to find the perfect way to eat.

Lauren became so fixated on calories and macros that she developed orthorexia, which can be described as healthy eating gone out of control. Steven Bratman, MD, first coined this term in his book *Health Food Junkies,* and defined it as "an obsession with eating only foods perceived to be of a certain status in terms of health, calories, or origin."[94] It is often extreme, where you are acutely critical of every single morsel you put into your mouth and don't put into your mouth. Lauren became terrified of certain foods and was consumed with only eating the very best of healthy things.[95]

Jason was still deployed at this time, and Lauren was so obsessed with calories, protein, fat, and carbohydrates that she avoided social situations. She became incapable of spending time with friends because she felt she wouldn't be able to eat. Her diet was that strict. But her cycle of bingeing continued as well. So when she wasn't being rigorous about her diet—she was bingeing like crazy. It became a vicious cycle of radical orthorexia and binge eating.

Then she found a woman who teaches intermittent fasting online. This method has you eating in a short window of time. For example, you fast between dinner and 12 pm the next day and then you eat all your food in a 6-hour period. So essentially you are fasting for 18 hours each day, from 6 pm until noon the next day.

---

94 [M26 Orthorexia Nervosa_July15.pdf – from IIN Module 26]. 2/3/2017 (accessed February 3, 2017).
95 2017. http://www.webmd.com/mental-health/eating-disorders/news/20001117/orthorexia-good-diets-gone-bad (accessed December 3, 2015).

The program came with a promise that if you fast 16–18 hours every day and sometimes fast for an entire 48-hour window—then you'll lose weight. Seems like a no-brainer. So Lauren bought the program and again, felt this was the answer! This was finally something that could keep the weight off for good. She felt this was something Jason could get on board with because he was into body building also, and it seemed like a good mix of diet and exercise.

The creator of the program encouraged bingeing behaviors as a perk of intermittent fasting, not realizing that it could be harmful to some of her customers. This caused Lauren's binge eating behaviors to spiral out of control. She would get home at 1 pm and have her first meal—which sometimes went on for hours. While at work, however, her brain wasn't functioning properly. She was so hungry and so tired that she couldn't think straight!

This was no way to go through life. She couldn't function at work. At this point Lauren started getting into podcasts and found someone named Maddy Moon who talked about freedom and never having to diet again. She touted the idea that there is no such thing as the perfect diet and that you don't have to be at war with your body. Along with these concepts, Maddy teaches people about letting go of control, learning how to not care what others think of you, self-love, breaking out of negative self-defeating patterns, and taking full control of your own life.[96]

---

96   "Home – Maddy Moon." 2017. *Maddy Moon.* http://maddymoon.com/ (accessed December 3, 2015).

It was the craziest concept Lauren had ever heard—not ever having to control your food intake. It wasn't dieting. It was about letting go of control of food. Completely!

Lauren told Jason about it and they were both a little terrified about what could happen. In the past, every time Lauren had let herself loose around food, she gained a bunch of weight quickly and it would spiral out of control. So naturally, they both thought this is what was going to happen.

Ever since Jason had told Lauren he had lost some of his attraction for her for gaining some weight, they struggled in their relationship. They had to consciously work through that issue. However, Lauren realized she needed to do this for herself—no matter the outcome. She told him, "I'm doing this for me and if you are no longer attracted to me because of this, I'm sorry but I need this for my mental health." She needed to let go and she needed to learn to accept herself.

There are so many synchronicities in life.

It's been over a year now, and not long after she found out about this freedom concept, she heard about the Institute for Integrative Nutrition (IIN) in another podcast. Lauren felt something immediately shift, and she dropped out of school right then and there and enrolled in the Health Coach Training Program at IIN. About halfway through the program at IIN there was an entire module focused on eating disorders, and one in particular sparked recognition in Lauren's mind. Binge Eating Disorder. She hadn't been able to put a name to this before. She didn't know this was a thing. But it is.

This is real. Binge Eating Disorder is a disease. It's not something that's in people's heads. It is an illness. What an eye-opener for Lauren. Learning about BED and realizing that this is what she was experiencing that entire time, all those years, was liberating.

So she let go of her control over food and allowed herself to eat what her body wanted. The first few months were a bit crazy, as she was eating a lot of things she hadn't let herself eat in a very long time. Lauren doesn't think she put on any weight, but she also stopped weighing herself. She did go through a few more binges but was eventually able to let go of the guilt. She got to where she refused to feel guilty or have shame around her binges.

Lauren allowed her behaviors to happen. If she was in the middle of a binge and felt that thing where she couldn't control it, like she wanted to stop but couldn't stop, Lauren simply let herself be in the binge. She learned to accept what was happening and accepted the emotions that came with it, in a nonjudgmental way. She would just go with it and continue to binge, but she would not feel guilty about it. A few months went by and the bingeing stopped.

The thought of bingeing again now does not sound appealing, even when Lauren is going through an emotional struggle. For example, a few months ago she and Jason almost broke up. It was a very difficult time for both of them. Instead of turning to food, however, for the first time, Lauren worked through her feelings. She called a friend and had her come over and they talked through it. Lauren was finally able to stop using food as a crutch.

Two life-changing books that helped Lauren move forward on this new healthy path were *Intuitive Eating: A Revolutionary Program That Works* by Evelyn Tribole, MS, RD, and *Health At Every Size: The Surprising Truth About Your Weight* by Linda Bacon, PhD. Both books and their associated movements focus on listening to your body and honoring its needs. Love yourself. Love yourself today—as you are right now.

This book is about moving beyond genetics and making choices to lead healthier lives—healthier than our parents and grandparents. This is true for Lauren as well. She remembers her mom dieting all her life and even taking diet pills. Growing up, Lauren watched her mom berate herself and struggle with her body. Sadly, she's still caught up in the diet/binge cycle and continues to feel insecure about her looks—despite the fact that Lauren sees her mom as absolutely gorgeous.

Unfortunately, she passed those insecurities on to Lauren by encouraging her to lose weight at a young age. Lauren's mom was the one who taught her how to lose weight. She would tell her things like "hide your body" and "don't wear a two-piece bathing suit." Lauren's sister has also struggled throughout much of her life with both anorexia nervosa and orthorexia nervosa. At one point, Lauren's sister did a colon cleanse and went raw vegan (while already being extremely thin), and her body shut down and started attacking itself by developing a huge rash from an autoimmune disorder. She is now totally on board with the non-dieting approach, and is focused on nourishing and accepting herself and being a good example for her three-year-old daughter. Thankfully, her skin has since healed. Thankfully, they listened to their bodies, learned about their mental struggles, and found a loving way to care for themselves.

Inspiration:

Lauren is very grateful to have endured the challenges she did around food and her body image, because now she can recognize the struggles in others and help set them free as well. She can relate to what they are going through because she lived it. If she told clients not to diet and just love your body without that understanding of where they are and what they've gone through, she wouldn't be the credible, inspirational coach she is today.

These experiences allowed Lauren to find her passion. She believes we all have a very specific purpose in this world, and her purpose is to help those suffering to love themselves. To teach them what radical self-acceptance feels like and how much it can change not only their lives, but the lives of those around them! We all strive to be happy and fulfilled in this life of ours, and Lauren's mission is to guide people in that direction. Her journey of struggling with body image and overcoming Binge Eating Disorder allows her to appreciate the gift of life.

Advice:

Life isn't meant to be perfect, and we aren't meant to feel amazing all the time. We grow the most from those moments of insecurity, sadness, discomfort, and despair. Lauren's advice to anyone going through a dark period is to just be in it.

"You *will* get through the pain; it won't last forever. Don't be afraid to just be with the pain, feel the discomfort, sit with the sadness ... for in those moments we are reminded of our true humanity. Trust that it will pass, and that there's an important lesson on the other side. Then when you are ready, stand up and take your next step forward."

Today, Lauren is a graduate of the Health Coach Training Program at IIN, and she instinctively reaches for foods that make her feel good. Like all of us, Lauren is not perfect. When she does eat something that doesn't make her feel great, she no longer beats herself up over it. She has released the guilt and her weight leveled off; she's back in the gym and feeling more mentally clear than she has ever felt before. Once she could put a label on what she had been experiencing her entire life, Lauren was set free. She feels like she is finally living life for the first time.

Contact:

Lauren loves to help people and is happy to schedule a free consultation. If you have been inspired by her story, feel free to contact Lauren at http://laurenkepler.com

Chapter 17

Carla: Eating Disorder and Stomach Issues

Good nutrition creates health in all areas of our existence. All parts are interconnected.

—*T. Colin Campbell*

Carla

Being the youngest of five children and an identical twin made Carla's early childhood years somewhat challenging, especially when trying to glean affection from her other siblings and even with friends. She and her twin sister always seemed to be competing with each other's personality and looks. It was a constant struggle for Carla growing up and sometimes still is today.

To make matters worse, towards the end of middle school Carla's parents were splitting up. Her dad had cheated on her mom after 30 years of marriage, and according to Carla, it was a pretty nasty divorce. As you can imagine, this also contributed to Carla's state of mind. Being a teenager with the additional stress of divorcing parents brings up all sorts of questions and internal chatter—things like where are we going to live, can we go to our friend's birthday party, can we have a sleepover, and even things like which parent is going to sign the form for school field trips. There was a lot of anxiety during that time—over and above the typical teen angst.

Carla didn't know it at the time, but because of all this stress she had developed stomach issues, which made it easier for her to cut back on eating. Every time she ate something that was too much or too spicy or too flavorful, it would upset her stomach badly. It was easier to cut back on meals because it made her stomach feel better when there was nothing in it. She had this constant fear that if she ate the wrong thing at the wrong time, she would get a horrible stomachache and feel ill the rest of the day or night.

In high school, food was a continual thought running through her mind—or rather the lack of it. It was easier not to eat, knowing if she didn't eat, there would be no stomachache. Carla would have a granola bar for breakfast and then not eat anything the entire day until she was back home.

During this time, Carla took a lot of advanced placement (AP) classes, which are essentially college-level courses taken in high school. She took as many of these as she could so that there wouldn't be as much of a financial burden on her parents when she went to college. Passing the associated exam for each AP course enabled Carla to get into a good college and receive college credit while still in high school, which ultimately saved on tuition.[97]

With all these AP courses came a lot of homework, and Carla often wouldn't be finished until 10 or 11 each night. She didn't want to eat dinner that late as it would have definitely upset her stomach. This schedule of hers made it easier and easier to avoid eating, and as she continued skipping dinner at night, Carla saw her body begin to change. This, she liked.

She felt great and thought she looked really good. Then she started to notice she was getting compliments on how much weight she had lost. She liked that also. Another thing Carla liked was that for the first time, she was standing out as being the skinny twin. Carla's sister wasn't overweight or even big for her size, but Carla enjoyed being labeled the skinny twin because for much of her early years she was the ugly twin.

Earlier on Carla had glasses while her sister didn't; Carla was more of an introvert and her sister was outgoing and had the popular friends. Carla mostly kept to herself. As she began getting compliments on how skinny she was, Carla took it as a sign of acceptance—the beauty factor. Now she was the pretty skinny twin. It wasn't her sister anymore—it was Carla!

That was high school. It was a pretty rough time for Carla and all her siblings because they kept moving from one house to another. The family's income drastically changed with the divorce, and that was an additional layer of stress. The main goal

---

97   2017. https://apstudent.collegeboard.org/exploreap/the-rewards (accessed November 27, 2015).

for Carla and her siblings was to get into a good college and to get as much financial aid as possible.

College was liberating. Even though Carla and her twin sister went to the same college, it was a very freeing experience. They were always very close. Even with the constant rivalry of who is the better one or the prettier one, they have always been very close. They always knew they wanted to go to college together. Still, it was a difficult time for the twins trying to figure out for themselves who they were by themselves without being by themselves. Each twin was trying to find herself. Oh, by the way, they were each clinically depressed.

They kind of knew something was wrong in high school, but they didn't actively seek out help. Once in college the twins helped each other find a psychiatrist, whom they saw separately. Carla was diagnosed with depression and anxiety, and her sister was diagnosed with depression. So along with all the other pressures of college life, they had depression to deal with.

Carla's diet in college fluctuated through various cycles of binge eating and binge drinking and then throwing up. She had gained between fifteen to twenty pounds and would get scared every time she ate too much, so she would make herself throw it up because she didn't want the calories. Carla, her sister, and their friends would try crazy diets for a day or two and then not follow through. They would hear of these diets through a friend of a friend. For example, someone heard of someone on the third floor who'd tried such-and-such diet, so the girls would try it. But they never seemed to stick with it long enough for it to work.

After college Carla and her sister moved to Washington, DC, and moved into an apartment together. Carla had a part-time job and a lot of free time, which she filled with exercise. A lot of exercise. She spent a lot of time browsing websites and reading blogs about different dietary strategies, looking for the latest health craze that she could try. Can you say "obsessed"?

She became fixated with fitness and health and tried many different diets, including diet pills. The pills, though, made her heart race and made her feel faint, so she would switch to another one. Then she tried a natural detox where for five days she would eat nothing but some green pills and some powder you were supposed to add to water. That particular diet lasted three days, until Carla found herself on the floor crying because she had no energy to do anything. She couldn't even get up. She didn't understand why she was doing this. It wasn't worth it. Carla hated herself for this.

When she finally had the energy to get up off the floor, Carla threw it all out. But then a week later, she found some-thing else and started another diet. She was spending all her spare time searching and researching diet fads and what the celebrities were doing to lose weight. Carla even had a Fitbit before they became popular. She became obsessed with track-ing every single thing that she ate. She would track everything down to a single piece of celery or a carrot stick.

It became so obsessive that Carla couldn't go out to a res-taurant to eat with friends or family because she wouldn't know what the calories were for a particular meal. She would have to guess; if she got the salad with pears and candied walnuts, how many calories were those? She would estimate the numbers as best as she could, but she was always stressed when she had to estimate the number of calories she had eaten. This was taxing on Carla emotionally and mentally. At the time she was at an okay weight, but not back to the weight she was in high school when she felt at her best.

During this time in DC, Carla was also exercising a lot and spending a lot of time walking around the neighborhood and jogging around the neighborhood. She was doing this two times every day. There were many times Carla went out to exercise right after she ate something because she wanted to negate the calories she had just consumed. She spent an inordinate amount of time writing down everything she ate into her food journal, matching it with exercise and keeping track of all sorts of numbers associated with her diet and exercise.

This went on for a few years up until about two years ago when Carla and her twin were moving out of the apartment they shared and into their own spaces. This was huge! They had lived together their entire lives up until this point—for approximately 26 years. Then two years ago they decided to move in with their respective boyfriends.

Boyfriends aside, this was an incredibly worrying time for Carla as she was in a job she hated and she felt that her twin, her other half, her best friend, was leaving her. At the time, her relationship with her boyfriend wasn't in the best place. They were fighting a lot, which added to Carla's anxiety.

Carla had no idea what her path was and she felt completely alone. She felt lost. She didn't know why she was here. She was in a very dark place and so alone. But, there was also a realization that she was tired of having these lonely thoughts and these feelings of being alone. She was sure that she couldn't be the only person this happened to. She didn't want a doctor to give her pills for depression or anxiety like they did when she was in college.

This was a turning point for Carla and she made a decision. She started researching wellness and alternative healing and found the Institute for Integrative Nutrition (IIN). After reading what it was all about, Carla knew instinctively that this was what she wanted to do. She felt a sense of hope and a feeling of belonging. Once enrolled in IIN, everything changed. She started to feel excited about this new adventure and immediately cleaned up her diet, and this led to a shift in her perspective about herself and her body image.

Going through IIN's Health Coach Training Program (HCTP) gave Carla a newfound love for food and got her excited about eating in a way she had never done before. She started focusing on foods that were good for her body instead of trying to get to a specific weight. She no longer gets stressed out over food. She doesn't have anxiety about how many calories or fat grams are in something she's eating. IIN taught her how to eat for her body, how to listen to her body. She now knows how to heal her stomach pains and she knows what her triggers are. Carla focuses on whole foods and healthy foods to stay away from her triggers. She also learned how to manage and help her stress and anxiety so she no longer wants to binge and throw up. Carla can now eat a meal without hating herself afterwards.

Carla is in a very different place than ever before. She has confidence in what she is doing; she has confidence in her likes and dislikes; she has confidence in herself. Even her personality has changed. Carla wakes up now and does things that amaze her to the point where she thinks, *Wow, Carla, you are awesome!* She is still humble and not conceited at all. She is just amazed at the kinds of things she does now that she never before had the confidence to do. Things she does for others; things she thinks of; things she creates.

Many people in Carla's life have no idea of some of the experiences she has gone through. Carla knows that there are other people out in the world who have gone through similar things. It has become her driving force—to seek out as many people as she can and help them understand that it's not as dark as things may seem. That they can get through this. To keep on pushing through and it will be worth it in the end.

Carla's diet changed drastically with each phase of her life. Back in high school she barely ate anything. Staples included cheese and crackers for lunch and dinner, mainly because she could easily count the calories and grams of fat. In college Carla ate crap. This included fast food and pizza, but then she would feel so guilty that she would try to throw it up. After college, she started eating more healthily and becoming more fit, and yet she was still consumed with the thought of counting calories, protein, carbs, fat, etc. So she would only eat those things for which she knew the numbers. Things like hummus, celery, carrots, and apples were standard fare. She also only ate what she considered snacks and never entire meals.

Today Carla has more balance in her diet. She eats green smoothies with almond milk, bananas, honey, and greens for breakfast. Snacks consist of granola bars and fruit. Lunch and dinner often involve quinoa and vegetables. Her boyfriend finds this boring, but Carla loves it because it's easy on her stomach and easy to digest.

She's learned how to balance everything in a way that works for her. Carla has found more of herself. She has found more of the likes she always knew were there but can now delve into more deeply. For example she has a passion for yoga, and it's become part of her life in a big way. In fact, two weeks after I interviewed Carla for this story, she was heading off to Hawaii to get her yoga teaching certification. She felt the calling and she's doing it. She never had the confidence to do anything like this before. There was always fear. Now there is hope, excitement, life.

Inspiration:

Despite all of the above, Carla knows that she would not be who she is today without having gone through all of these experiences. She believes that things happen to nudge us, or sometimes outright push us, in the right direction. Carla doesn't regret any experiences she's had, good or bad—even the most difficult dark ones. Those experiences gave her the motivation and inspiration to help herself and others. She wouldn't be where she is today if it weren't for those hard times.

Advice:

Carla's advice to anyone going through a difficult time is this: don't give up. Know that you are not alone and that you are loved. She understands that hearing these words is difficult because often people do feel alone and unloved. Even when people hear the words, they don't believe it. She understands this because she was there. It was difficult for Carla to believe things like this that she heard or read. She always thought she was alone and the only person going through this. However, it simply wasn't and is not true.

Understanding this now, Carla wishes people would reach out more. Reach out to others who may have similar problems or issues. Learn from each other. Motivate each other to keep pushing forward. Once she began to heal, Carla found out that millions of other people were going through what she had. This made her feel more powerful and motivated to keep pushing through and to help others who need it. Don't give up! You are worthy of love and greatness, and we are all here to help.

Contact:

Carla is a Holistic Health Coach from the Institute for Integrative Nutrition, dedicated to educating clients in making healthy choices while providing support on goals they develop themselves to improve their overall well-being. She is passionate about living an authentic life and wants to share her experiences, passions, and knowledge with others so they may do the same for themselves! She is also a certified yoga teacher (RYT-200) and teaches the importance of movement and breath to reduce stress and to promote balance in all areas of life.

If you've been inspired by Carla's story and would like to contact her, please visit her website or send e-mail: http://www.tribeofwell-being.com/, bica.morgan@gmail.com

Chapter 18

Lisa: Eating Disorder and Self-Esteem

You are allowed to be both a masterpiece and
a work in progress simultaneously.

—Sophia Bush

Lisa

Lisa's story also begins back in her childhood. At a very young age she manifested a deep psychological issue with her body image, emanating from an incident with her sister. Lisa was three when nine-year-old Sheri challenged her to a race, Lisa riding a bicycle against Sheri running. Being on foot, Sheri was able to cut through all the lawns and poor Lisa had to go all the way around. You can see how this ended. It was totally unfair. But three-year-old Lisa wanted to impress her older sister so much, she rode her little heart out. When it was over, her sister sang her a song about the difference between fat and thin.

Fat and skinny had a race all around the steeplechase.
Fat fell down and broke her face and skinny won the race.

Being a child herself, Sheri had no idea of the negative impact and humiliation this simple rhyme would have, but Lisa remembers that song to this day. It's been like an anchor weighing her down. If you're fat you lose. If you're thin you win. Wow! What a life lesson for a three-year-old to learn. Unbeknownst to Lisa at the time, it had a huge impact on her life.

On the positive side, it instilled in her a love of health and fitness. In her mid-forties now, Lisa has been exercising since the age of ten and became a personal trainer at nineteen. Health and fitness were so much a part of who she was and is, that she wanted to help others work out and get fit. Growing up she was consistently within a normal range for weight and body size for her age, but on the negative side, she always felt weighed down. There was always that three-year-old voice telling her *fat equals loser*. This internal message made it impossible for Lisa to see herself as others did. No matter how fit she was in reality, her vision of herself was as a big girl, and this distorted body image hindered her ability to be happy.

With the self-perception of being big, Lisa always felt it was a struggle to keep her weight down. She started making up her own rules of what she could and couldn't eat. These rules changed with the wind. One week she would only eat the crust of pizza; another week she gave up ketchup. When she was a little older, she used herbal pills to speed up her metabolism. For six years! During college, Lisa focused on all the fat-free stuff that flooded the market, thinking that was the answer. Like the rest of us, she didn't realize those no-fat and low-fat things (I can't call food) were loaded with sugar and chemicals. We all know now that doesn't work and only makes things worse. She also tried the Paleo diet for a while, but felt awful and even gained weight!

As a brief aside, the Paleo diet or lifestyle is based on hundreds of thousands of years of human evolution. Back before we had agriculture, humans lived on real, whole unprocessed foods, going back about 200,000 years. Agriculture has only been around for approximately 10,000 years, which is not enough time for our bodies to adapt to eating things like wheat and sugar. Paleo enthusiasts vary in their diet, but staples include grass-fed meats, wild-caught fish, and vegetables. Some eat dairy and others sometimes enjoy things like bread and rice, though it's not typical.

As she progressed through these experiments with diet, Lisa also explored cutting carbohydrates out of her regimen, which then led to a variety of fasts and cleanses. One of these was the lemonade cleanse. This was a three-day fast where you ingested nothing except water, lemon juice, and maple syrup. She liked the results so much that a new rule emerged: every Friday would be lemon-fast day. This went on for almost a year until some medical issues began to emerge. At the time she didn't realize it, but an MRI showed that she had severely irritated her entire digestive tract with this cleanse. Medication was prescribed to reverse the effects of her acute acid reflux, and as you might imagine, eating became tremendously uncomfortable. Lisa had been so obsessed with her distorted self-image that she stopped thinking about her overall health and focused only on how she looked.

Acid reflux happens when stomach acids find their way up into the esophagus, causing heartburn. There are a variety of triggers, including being overweight, smoking, drinking alcohol, and even certain foods like tomatoes and citrus. The best way to treat acid reflux is to lose weight, eat smaller meals, don't eat 2–3 hours before bedtime, stop smoking, and try propping up your pillow by five inches or so. If you must, take an antacid, but realize that prolonged use over time can lead to other complications.[98]

It's fairly common for those obsessed with body image to turn to the fitness industry for comfort. Lisa was no different. After she became a certified fitness specialist, she later went on to become a licensed massage therapist, triathlon coach, and health and lifestyle motivator. She fueled her fixation on maintaining the perfect body image by helping others maintain theirs. She also developed a fascination with fitness contests, including racing, endurance sports, and figure competitions. Over a period of about twenty years, Lisa became a health and fitness guru and role model. People looking in from the outside would see a self-motivated inspirational woman who was a leader in her chosen profession.

What they didn't see was the scared three-year-old hanging on by a thread, terrified of gaining even one ounce. She described it as being a prisoner within herself, always having to

---

98 Cold, Flu & Cough, Eye Health, Heart Disease, Pain Management, Sexual Conditions, Skin Problems, and Sleep Disorders et al. 2017. "What Is Acid Reflux Disease?" Webmd. http://www.webmd.com/heartburn-gerd/guide/what-is-acid-reflux-disease?page=3.

maintain the perfect figure because it was expected of her. For example, leading up to the day of a figure competition, Lisa would starve herself! Typically, judges were looking for muscularity and symmetry among other things, and most women have a layer of body fat over their muscle, which hides definition. Lisa felt that the last-minute starving would allow her muscles to shine through.

She carried around this feeling of self-loathing. Lisa described to me that she had no escape from her inner demons. There was no hiding from her ego telling her how horrible she was. She literally beat herself up every day. When she was thin, it was a good day. When she felt fat or bloated, it was a bad day; she was bad, a loser. Lisa was damaging her body, her mind, and her soul. Even on those days when she was thin and felt good, there was always that voice in her head telling her things like, my stomach could be flatter, or I need to lose two more pounds. Nothing was ever good enough. She was never good enough.

Growing up, Lisa always seemed to have hips and a butt, even back in elementary school, while all the other little girls had stick figures. Then she went through puberty early, like in fourth grade, so she started developing much earlier than the other girls around her. Lisa had an image of herself that she was an ogre. That three-year-old voice in her head was always present. At one point as a teenager, she even tried to be bulimic, but could never actually make herself throw up. She tried and tried and tried, but just couldn't do it and laughed it off as poor gag reflexes. Throughout her early years, Lisa went through various phases such as only eating lettuce. One phase had her drinking a gallon of water every day, which went on for years to the point that she got bloated and distended. Like pictures we've all seen of poor, malnourished children whose bellies are extended beyond their natural circumference. She finally realized she was hurting herself, and with this revelation recognized other periods in her life that were hurtful and not helpful.

There was an entire series of unhealthy behaviors that took years to recognize. One of those was binge eating. As with most people with Binge Eating Disorder (BED), this was a private thing. Lisa reflected that her BED began back in high school. If there was a cake in the house, she would take a sliver. Then go back ten minutes later for another forkful. Then later, it was back for another bite or two. Soon the entire cake was gone. She couldn't help herself. But she could go to the gym and try to undo all those calories with hours of exercise. This too became a pattern. On the way home from the gym after a monster 2-hour workout, Lisa would stop at the store for a box of low-calorie cookies. Remember the private part? She would eat the entire box of cookies in her car, stop at the gas station to throw away the box, and then go home as if it had never happened. This behavior occurred two or three times each week and continued throughout her life. To this day Lisa stays vigilant, continually on the lookout for triggers to this downward spiral.

Fortunately, her obsession with fitness never wavered, and in ways this balanced her binge eating. She ventured into the world of endurance sports and found peace in long-distance running. Lisa ran half marathons, marathons, and even ultra-marathons (defined as any foot race longer than a traditional 26.2 miles of a marathon), which ultimately led to a fascination with triathlons. Defined as a multi-sport endurance event, triathlons include a swim, a bicycle ride, and a run, all of varying lengths. The gold standard of triathlons is the Ironman, which is 140.6 miles broken out in a 2.4-mile swim, a 112-mile bike ride, and a full marathon at 26.2 miles. Lisa, to her credit, has completed approximately 50 triathlons,[99] including 2 full Ironman triathlons.[100]

Training for long-distance races took Lisa out of the real world. She was comfortable being alone and enjoyed the feeling of movement. She called it "moving meditation." Each new race was an irresistible thrill. Reflecting back, though, Lisa realized that racing was feeding her eating disorder. It all goes back to the same song she heard at the age of three. Everything stemmed back to that song. It never left her. If she raced well, she was good. If she didn't, she was bad. Training for good races became another obsession. It kept her moving and distracted her from facing the truth. Subconsciously she thought if she worked out religiously, she could somehow make up for the times she binged.

For 27 years Lisa kept up appearances. To the outside world, she was the epitome of health. She had coached and trained people in all levels of fitness, in triathlons, health and lifestyle management, running and weight loss. She helped thousands of people attain their health and fitness goals.

99   "ULTRA Running Races & Resources | Ultramarathonrunning.Com." 2017. *Ultramarathonrunning.Com.* http://www.ultramarathonrunning.com/ (accessed March, 2017).
100 2017. *IRONMAN.Com.* http://www.ironman.com/ (accessed January 25, 2017).

Somewhere along the line, though, she recognized that there was more to fitness than exercise and controlling food intake. Lisa had an epiphany that helping people had little to do with fixing bad habits and everything to do with their lack of happiness. It was time for a change.

Lisa described her life as a "journey of fear, always worrying about her weight and what people thought of her." She recognizes now that this had driven her. Fear of not having certain things so that she could have this figure she worked so hard for. The image she created for herself with her body is something Lisa has ownership of. But it also owns her. There is no room to gain weight. If she gained an ounce on her belly, then she was worthless. For a few years, Lisa never ate in a restaurant. Not one morsel. If she happened to go out with friends, she would eat before going to the restaurant. While not quite a diet, it's also not very socially acceptable. She had restricted herself so much that having a piece of pizza was not an option. It just didn't happen. This scenario describes orthorexia, which is taking healthy eating to an extreme. When Lisa learned about this, it brought about a new way of thinking. She realized she wasn't doing herself any favors by being that regimented and rigid.

At forty-two she reached a breaking point. Lisa knew she couldn't maintain this absurd and abusive (as she called it) lifestyle anymore. She was exhausted and somehow defeated by her own successes. She made a decision that would change her life and enrolled in the Health Coach Training Program at the Institute for Integrative Nutrition (IIN). It was during this intensive yearlong program that Lisa heard the terms Binge

Eating Disorder and orthorexia for the first time. Lisa had never actually labeled herself as having an eating disorder. It was eye opening to say the least. Learning about various eating disorders and being able to understand them and what triggers them gave her the clarity she needed around her own eating issues. Being able to put a name to what she had been experiencing all these years was somewhat liberating for her. As she related this story, she said it all comes down to body image and self-confidence. This enabled her to make some huge lifestyle changes. She learned to express her feelings in a more authentic way. She stopped racing and she modified her diet in ways that are healthful rather than obsessive.

Lisa began to look at food as nourishment, as nutrients, as healing medicine rather than as something she needed to control. She began exploring the concept of clean eating, which for her meant only eating foods that add nutritional value and health to the body. She even started a Facebook group called Keep It Clean with a focus on health. She solicited friends to the group and now has thirty members who interact with each other, learning how to eat clean and take care of themselves. Lisa had an ulterior motive, however, and these thirty people became her support team. They helped her push through her torment on a daily basis.

Each and every day, without fail, Lisa dedicated time to write something motivational in the group about health and wellness. She made this decision to write every day for a full year, thinking that as she healed herself she would be helping others heal as well. This practice helped Lisa in more ways than she could have imagined. She recognized that she is not alone, and with the support of her thirty cohorts, she began to heal. As did all thirty people in the group. They confessed their bad habits and negative behaviors, they asked questions and found answers, and they learned about their own issues, emotional and mental. They healed together. Lisa is eternally grateful for this group and for what they did for each other throughout that year. Lisa told me, "One of the most profound things I learned from leading this group is that asking for help isn't a sign of weakness, sitting alone in silence is."

It's amazing how our minds work. This year, on Lisa's forty-fourth birthday, her mother related a story to her, saying, "Oh Lisa, 44 years ago today I was in so much pain because you were so big. They couldn't get you out of me. You were so big and had these broad shoulders." Wow!!! Lisa heard this story every year of her life on what was supposed to be a happy occasion. Is it any wonder she had issues with her body size? She had never thought about this before, but after she got off the phone with her mother she realized that every time her mom said the word "big," Lisa felt like a nail was being driven into her chest.

Prior to this, Lisa had never connected the dots. She had never thought about it before. Lisa doesn't blame her mom at all. She didn't know any better; she was experiencing something for herself and merely telling her story from her perspective. It was her mom's story, not Lisa's. But, Lisa owned that story. That little girl inside of her decided somewhere along the line that she was fat, that she was ugly, and that she didn't deserve to be happy.

Life is very different for Lisa today. She graduated from the Institute for Integrative Nutrition (IIN) in September of 2016 and has never felt freer. She has come to terms with her reality and decided to enroll in life-coaching courses with "Your Infinite Life" to help her explore her early childhood. This program "serves as a bridge for people as they are guided to discover, honor and live their unique life's purpose." Lisa now has an entirely new outlook on life. Her perspective is that nothing is about weight loss anymore; it's all about life gain.[101]

She also understands that she is still healing and probably will be for the rest of her life. She knows her lifelong fears stemmed back to her childhood, and the reason she suffered so much internally for most of her life is because she never faced the feelings from her past. Lisa told me, "the heart breaks open, not closed." She was carting around open wounds that were never going to heal until she felt them. It's been a long road, but her wounds are beginning to heal. She feels like she was a superstar at protecting herself from sadness, but now she is a *rock* star at facing it!

Never judge a book by its cover. So many times in our society, people are judged by appearances. By how they look, the car they drive, the house they own, the clothes they wear, their speech patterns, etc. Yet, often, the most seemingly fit and healthy among us are the ones who need the most help. They are the ones with low self-esteem, guilt, judgment, and insecurity issues. For Lisa, food and exercise were her drugs

---

101 "Course Overview: Your Infinite Life." 2017. *Yourinfinitelifeonline.Com*. https://www. yourinfinitelifeonline.com/courses.php (accessed March 14, 2017).

of choice, her addiction. Thankfully, she is able to use her journey and what she learned through her experiences to help others. She looks forward to helping many more people as she continues to heal herself.

Lisa is grateful to be a part of this book. She will write her own someday, but for now just getting her story out there is enough. She wanted to thank you all deeply for reading her story, and she hopes it finds its way into the universe to help whomever is ready.

Inspiration:

Lisa believes health is our birthright. Taking ownership of her rights and deciding where to draw the line for her boundaries has literally changed her life. We all have a story, but when we choose to bury our story, it metastasizes like a cancer. It will infect you and all those around you. Facing your truth may seem frightening. Lisa used to think that as well, but she discovered something even more frightening: facing your denials. She used to think she was superhuman. She thought she didn't need anyone. She used to pride herself in going at it alone. Then one day she broke and there was no one to save her from herself. This awakening revealed a vulnerability she had no idea existed. Lisa is eternally grateful for all of her suffering, for without it, she wouldn't be who she is today. For the first time in her life she likes who she is, and she's not ashamed to admit it.

Advice:

Darkest moments are the toughest because you no longer recognize yourself. This is when mistakes are made, accidents happen, and the most punishing behavior takes place. For Lisa, exercise was always her savior. As much as she abused it, it gave her perspective and hope. Knowing what she knows now, Lisa's advice for when you are in your darkest moments is to seek out the most positive thing you can. Take what you are feeling and enter it into your search engine, then read the quotes, watch the Ted Talks, and listen to the podcasts. Knowing that you are not alone may give you comfort. Knowing there are others feeling similar things allows you to understand there are options.

Lisa also shared this:

Victor Frankel writes it best in *A Man's Search for Meaning*. Frankel says, "Everything can be taken from a man but one thing; the last of the human freedoms—to choose one's attitude in any given set of circumstances, to choose one's own way."

This gives me hope that whatever I am feeling at the moment is my choice. That means that I am always in control of myself, therefore if I am in control of my sadness, I can also be in control of my happiness.

Contact:

Lisa is a graduate of IIN, a Life Coach at Your Infinite Life Coaching Company, a Licensed Massage Therapist MA 32314, USAT Triathlon Coach Level 1, Personal Fitness Trainer, and Innovative Body Solutions Trainer. As a health coach, Lisa offers clients across the country an opportunity to discover their own simple truths. She is honored to share a part of your journey. You can contact Lisa for a free health-coaching session or information on any of her services at www.lisa-callahan.com or www.trilifebody.com

Chapter 19

Jess: Weight and Crippling Menstrual Cramps

*Find something you adore that happens
to be good for you, that's how you live
long healthy lives.*

—*Dr. Oz*

Jess

In a previous life, Jess was a funeral director. How often do you hear that? While in this role she got pregnant with twins, and though she was able to return to work part-time, after giving birth, her full-time position was no longer available to her. Around this same time an acquaintance was opening up a weight loss center. Jess had about fifty pounds to lose, so she stopped by to see what it was all about. The acquaintance was way too busy to chat with her, and as way of an apology mentioned she needed to hire someone. Jess flippantly responded that she had just given her two-week notice and was hired on the spot!

This began Jess's journey as a weight loss counselor. It also kicked off her personal journey with health and wellness. At the time, Jess knew nothing about how to help others with their weight loss, but she jumped right into this family-owned business. She described it as a similar structure as LA Weight Loss—high protein, low carb. They use one-on-one counseling and personalized sessions focused on healthy eating habits.

Jess saw her clients twice each week in a factory-style setting. In other words, she met with clients for fifteen minutes, then they were off and she was meeting with her next client. So she met with four clients per hour. This was interesting to her; you had about fifteen minutes to meet a person, build rapport, take a look at their food diary, offer suggestions, and help plan meals, motivate them, and send them on their way. Wow! That's a lot for fifteen minutes!

It became an exciting challenge for Jess and she found her passion. She dove into it and learned as much as she could while on the job and off. Ultimately she got to a point where she felt she needed more. Jess would get to a certain point with her clients and be stuck. She didn't know where else to go. She was at a loss as to how to help them further. She wished for a roadmap or for someone to show her the direction.

This led to Jess seeking out and researching various certifications and online programs, which brought her to the Institute for Integrative Nutrition. IIN's Health Coach Training Program immediately resonated with Jess. She enrolled, went through the entire program, and completed it last year while still working at the weight loss center two days per week. She had a lot of momentum while going through the yearlong program at IIN, and even worked with four different clients as a health coach during that time. Now, though, she misses the structure and accountability of the program.

It's interesting how often I hear that all coaches have coaches. It's no different for Jess. She feels like she has stalled, and she's at the point where she is considering finding her own health coach to help motivate her and keep her accountable to her goals and dreams. Jess feels having a health coach in her corner will help her get her momentum back.

Through her time working at the weight loss center, Jess released fifty pounds. That experience coupled with the IIN curriculum guided her on a journey of self-discovery. She learned a lot about herself. One interesting thing she discovered after giving birth to her second set of twins was that every time she ovulated, she dropped two eggs. Not wanting a third set of twins, Jess had a tubal ligation along with her C-section.

Since the tubal ligation, Jess's menstruation cycles have been extremely painful, so she started experimenting with food to see how certain foods manifested in her physically and emotionally. She began a 21-day elimination diet. Elimination diets are used in many ways, such as to detox, reset cravings, and to discover food sensitivities or allergies. They are all slightly different depending on one's goals. For example, some elimination diets exclude corn, soy, dairy, gluten, and eggs for three weeks, and then you add in one of those over a three-day period to see if it has any impact. Then you add the others, each one separately, over a three-day period.

Others exclude coffee and alcohol as well. Some go further and have you avoid any forms of sugar. Jess's version had her eating only nuts, seeds, fruits, vegetables, and oils for 21 days, and tea instead of coffee. She learned a lot in those three weeks. The first two days she described as crippling. She had pains in places she never would have expected, like down her leg. She's not a big pill taker, but at times she had to take something for the pain. Jess understood that this was something her body had to go through if she wanted to learn about any food sensitivities. These pains are part of the detox process the body goes through; almost like withdrawals.

During this process, Jess had her period—but the amazing thing was that she never felt bloated and never had any cramps. This was astounding to her! Talk about self-discovery. Jess realized that she herself had been causing that pain with her food choices. Let me repeat that: she was self-inflicting pain with the food she was eating.

This was about a year ago, and it was a wake-up call for Jess. It was an eye-opener. It raised some curiosity as to what had been causing her pain. In her version of the elimination diet, Jess excluded almost everything! Now it was time to add foods back into her diet one at a time to see what effect they had. Jess added one food at a time over the period of a month. The first month she added coffee back into her regimen. She experienced slight cramping, but not severe, and it was good to know that coffee contributed to her pain.

The second month, Jess added dairy, which definitely caused some bloating and pain for her. The following month, she added grains. Grains caused her mild discomfort and a little bloating, but not too bad that she couldn't handle it. Through her self-experimentation, Jess discovered that dairy and coffee had the biggest impact in terms of bloating and cramping—around the time of her periods. This is amazing! She now knows what foods to avoid and at what times. She understands what triggers pain and bloating in her body. Armed with this knowledge, Jess can live her life without wondering if something she eats will trigger discomfort.

Once you have a successful experiment and understand the results, it's easy to keep going. Not that I'm recommending anyone avoid doctors—they are necessary. However, at times it can be fascinating and satisfying to discover things about your own body on your own. This is something taught in the Health Coach Training Program at IIN: how to work with clients to encourage and motivate and help them towards self-healing. With one success under her belt, Jess embraced this concept, and any time she feels discomfort she has the knowledge to move forward and try to figure it out.

For example, Jess was experiencing chronic pain in the heel of her foot and did some research. Without any blood work, she came to the possibility that she might be lacking magnesium. She had all the symptoms. So, Jess started taking supplements and reduced her coffee intake. She found that drinking a lot of coffee could deplete magnesium. These changes helped her and her heels are now free of pain.

There is a lot of self-discovery going on in her life, which is the sign of a good coach. Having an understanding of how things work in one's own body and having self-compassion and self-love are qualities that make one a good health coach. If you've experienced things for yourself, you are better equipped to help guide others through similar events.

Jess is now trying to find doctors to work with so that she can share her health coach skills. This is proving difficult, though, because many doctors find it easier or more familiar to work with medications as opposed to nutrition. We, as health coaches, have heard many times that nutrition is not something taught in medical school, at least not to any great extent. Unfortunately, doctors are sometimes bound by practices forced upon them by the insurance and pharmaceutical worlds.

While she is seeking work, Jess continues to spread the word to friends and family that we are what we eat. She still works two days per week at the weight loss center that helped her release fifty pounds. However, the practices the center uses to help people are no longer in alignment with her beliefs. Through her studies at IIN and with her own self-discovery, Jess understands more about how nutrition is a bio-individual thing. There is no one-size-fits-all solution. This is causing some internal struggles as she finds herself in conflicting positions. At times when she is consulting with clients, she will say, "Well, the center recommends this, but you know that with nutrition there is never concrete evidence to that recommendation because no two bodies are the same." She is toeing the company line yet encouraging people to realize they are unique and that their body may need something a little more or different.

Today, Jess enjoys a wide-ranging diet including meat, although much less than she used to eat. She has limited her animal protein intake and is very cautious of her sources of protein. She excludes all soy, for example, as most soy is processed and genetically modified. Jess also reads ingredient labels very carefully. She still eats dairy, but again, not as much as she used to. For example, she used to eat yogurt twice per day. Now she avoids yogurt and only has kefir once in a while, which contains more probiotics than regular yogurt (which are helpful bacteria that keep your gut healthy).[102]

Her diet is very low in grains as she says, "Carbs definitely stick to me." As opposed to fruits and vegetables, which play a very large role in her diet. She tries to keep things as simple as possible, and creates meals with few ingredients. But, she still has a sugar addiction that she doesn't think she'll ever quite kick. Her twins are now four and seven—so Halloween is a challenge. Jess said she gave away two-and-a-half-gallon-sized bags of candy to friends and family, and there is still a ton of candy in her house.

Jess has been able to maintain the fifty-pound weight loss, for the most part. A few weeks ago, though, she realized she's up about ten pounds in the past two years. It was a bit of a slap in the face for her, but Jess understands that this is how it happens. A couple or five pounds each year, and over time it adds up. Ten pounds doesn't come on overnight, and it doesn't go away overnight. These types of experiences also make us better health coaches.

---

102 "Is Soy Bad for You? – Dr. Axe." 2017. *Dr. Axe.* https://draxe.com/is-soy-bad-for-you/ (accessed April 30, 2017).

Jess turned to the MyFitnessPal app, which helps her understand her caloric intake and output.[103] It's a great app to use to keep track of all the food one eats on a daily basis. You can enter goals in terms of calories, protein, carbohydrates, fat, fiber, etc., as well as some micronutrients such as saturated fat, trans fat, cholesterol, sugar, calcium, and iron. It's been shown that keeping a food diary helps people lose more weight than those who don't track their food. Daily food journals help keep you accountable and aware of your intake. Additionally it tracks calorie output, meaning exercise.

Along with this app, Jess bought a program called VFX Body, which is a 12-week diet and exercise program designed specifically for women. The premise behind John Barban's program is that women should never diet like men. Our bodies are different and require different levels of nutrients, calories, etc.[104]

The VFX Body program recommended three workouts per week for Jess. Alas, she is an all-or-nothing kind of person; so three workouts per week just didn't work for her. She is the type of person who was used to exercising six days per week for at least an hour at a time. With four young children at home, it became difficult to get in six one-hour workouts each week. So Jess being all or nothing would go back to the nothing end of the spectrum.

Knowing this, when Jess began this program six weeks prior to our interview, she went in with a different mindset.

---

103 "Free Calorie Counter, Diet & Exercise Journal | Myfitnesspal.Com." 2017. *Myfitnesspal. Com.* http://www.myfitnesspal.com/ (accessed January 25, 2017).
104 "VFX BODY." 2017. *Vfxbody.Com.* http://www.vfxbody.com/learn-more/ (accessed January 27, 2017).

She focused on keeping in mind that this is not a chore, that she enjoyed this, and if she could get in three days each week— that's awesome. If there were weeks where she only exercised one day, that's okay too! She picks up right where she left off. Now Jess is definitely in this differently. In the past she would try to only focus on diet and not exercise. She said she hated exercise. Today, her mindset has shifted to a more balanced perspective of physical activity.

Her recommendation to anyone in a similar situation is to find a form of exercise that you love. Also replace the word *exercise* with *activity*. Think back to when you were a child: what did you love to do when you were younger? Don't think of it as exercise or as a chore or as something you "have to" do or "should do." Reflecting on the activities you truly enjoyed as a child is great advice when seeking a form of physical activity you'll stick with. Because let's face it: if you don't enjoy it, you are going to stop doing it.

Jess always keeps this in mind and it is helpful for her. She's doing things she loved as a child so exercise is no longer a chore. For example, in her yard they have a slack line. Jess described it as a kind of tightrope that you hang between two trees. It's a bit slacker (thus the name) and has more give or bounce than a tightrope. At first, she couldn't even stay on it for more than a second. But Jess kept at it and now she can stand on it. That's progress!

Instead of going off by herself to work out, now she grabs her kids and they all go for a bike ride together. Roller-skating is another thing she does with her kids. Jess loved roller-skating when she was young, so being able to do it with her children is both fun and a blessing. She enjoys being active with her children! And she gets to see their joy in doing these things with her. This is beautiful—her kids will grow up with an active, healthy mom who loves spending time with them. They will be happier and healthier, and their children will be happier and healthier. What a legacy to pass down!

Inspiration:

Jess is grateful for her journey, as it taught her how to truly communicate with others and really listen. In the past, she was just waiting for her next chance to talk or to give her opinion. She didn't really focus on what the other person was saying. She's grown so much through her experiences, and her relationships have improved greatly, especially with her husband. She says communicating is a bit easier now. She's learned self-care and self-love. And most importantly, Jess has created awareness not only with food, but with gratitude and humility.

Advice:

Jess's advice for others going through difficult times is to focus on just one minute. Just get through the next minute. Concentrate on deep breathing for one minute. Allow this one minute to be grounding. Think about the good things in life, the beautiful things in the universe. Focus on that. Release the negativity.

When she feels down, Jess focuses on her eating. She says that food is information. I love that! She also says:

"If I am fueling my body with junk, I tend to feel depressed, sluggish, bloated, and foggy. To get myself out of that vicious cycle—of feel like crap *equals* eat crap, eat crap *equals* feel like crap—I eliminate processed food and focus on raw vegetables and fats. My body responds best to high-quality fats (nuts, avocados, MCT oil, and coconut oil), raw vegetables, and berries. When I'm in a 'funk' I know that's not normal for me, so it is very important for me to journal. I journal my food (good and bad), my goals for the day, and my gratitude. It is a great 'go-to' tool I use as needed. Sometimes we just need little reminders, and my journaling is my reminder of how great life truly is."

Contact:

Today, Jess is an Integrative Nutrition Health Coach using what she learned at IIN and her own life experiences to help others overcome health issues. If you want to learn more, contact Jessica Tarleton, INHC at 570-527-2572 or send her an email at evolvinghealthandwellness@gmail.com

Chapter 20

Deb: Losing 100 Pounds

The body achieves what the mind believes.

—Anonymous

Deb

Deb is forty-seven years young, 5'3", and weighs 137 pounds. These stats are important to her as we'll see later in her story. She is a certified fitness trainer, a triathlon coach, a nutrition coach, and a registered nurse. While I was interviewing her for this book, Deb was in her car on the way to become certified by the Road Runner's Club of America (RRCA) to add "running coach" to her repertoire.

Specializing in strength, nutrition, and multi-sport coaching, Deb started a company called 3TimesFitness. She is still a surgical nurse part-time and may never give that up as she spent so much time and effort studying to become a nurse. She has an extensive medical background having worked in ICU (Intensive Care Unit), CCU (Critical Care Unit), and was a certified diabetic educator. Becoming a coach, though, has always been a dream of hers, so starting her company six months ago was the beginning of a dream come true.

Her love for people and coaching was the impetus for her moving forward in this direction. She's now the head trainer for a group called Friends in Training, which focuses on half and full marathon training. Deb also coaches people in the gym for strength work, and she coaches triathletes who are seeking to improve in various levels of triathlons.

Personally, Deb has completed 26 full marathons. A marathon, for those who don't know, is 26.2 miles. She has also run numerous half marathons (13.1 miles) and tons of smaller races. Deb began her running career in 2005 and did her first triathlon in 2010. Since that time she completed four full Ironman triathlons. Wow! I'm impressed.

For the record, a triathlon is a multi-sport endurance event. They include a swim, a bicycle ride, and a run of varying lengths, with no breaks between. In other words, you swim first, then jump on your bike and let the airflow dry you off until it's time to run. There is very little time to transition between these events. The gold standard of triathlons is the Ironman, which is 140.6 miles broken out in a 2.4-mile swim, a 112-mile bike ride, and a full marathon at 26.2 miles. I'm exhausted just writing that.[105]

Deb is an Ironman athlete. Along with her four full Ironman competitions, she has also completed nine half-Ironmans and

---

105 2017. *IRONMAN.Com*. http://www.ironman.com/ (accessed January 25, 2017).

numerous smaller ones. She currently does CrossFit and a lot of strength training. CrossFit is a trademarked fitness regimen developed by Greg Glassman that incorporates "constantly varied functional movements performed at high intensity."[106] The functional movements are taken from a variety of disciplines such as gymnastics, running, weightlifting, rowing, etc. Essentially, when doing CrossFit, you are doing intense work in a short amount of time, which leads to dramatic gains in overall fitness.

While building muscle and strength are important, even critical for athletes, Deb is a big believer that these things can help everyone in their everyday life. She lives this lifestyle and trains others in this lifestyle. She calls this "living a dream come true."

She also says that timing is everything. Deb's nursing job is very flexible and allows her the time to be able to do these other things, which feed her soul. She was able to cut back more in her nursing job and take on more in her coaching business. Today she is a full-time coach and does nursing a few days per month.

Deb has been married for twenty-five years and has two children. One is twenty-one and the other fourteen; both have participated in running events, including triathlons for the oldest. Her husband also does CrossFit, is a runner, and has done triathlons as well. It's become a family affair and a lifestyle they all enjoy together.

---

106 "Crossfit: Forging Elite Fitness: Sunday 170514." 2017. Crossfit.Com. http://www.crossfit.com (accessed January 25, 2017).

Flashback ... Deb has been heavy her entire life. She told me she was a chubby kid, a heavy teen, and a heavy adult. She was even heavy when she got married. Deb has no stories that start out, "When I was young and could wear a size two." Or, "I wish I could fit back into my wedding dress." Her story is a little backwards but in a good way. Deb *never* wants to fit back into her wedding gown, as it was a size 21 and today she wears a size four. She is much smaller now than ever in her life. Well, other than being an infant and toddler, of course.

Deb was always heavy, but she had a great life. She was never one to sit in a corner hiding from the world. She always had a big personality and a big presence. She had a lot of friends and a lot of boyfriends. Deb knew how to enjoy life even though she wasn't one of the thin girls. She didn't know how to sit on the sidelines and was in band, on the flag team, and even did gymnastics, as she says, as a "little fat kid." She didn't let anything hold her back from enjoying life. She liked doing a variety of things even if she wasn't good at them and even if she wasn't in good shape. It didn't matter. She always tried and she always enjoyed them. She always enjoyed life.

This is why she has a very strong belief today that you can do anything. You can always try. There is always something you can do to work towards a better life. She doesn't like it when she hears clients say things like, "I have bad knees so I can't do anything." Yes, you can! There is always something you can do. Okay, so maybe you won't be running any marathons with those knees, but you can swim.

Being heavy most of her life left Deb trying various things to lose the weight, such as Weight Watchers, which she says she tried 10,000 times. It was the typical story, though: she would lose some then gain it back, then lose some then gain it back again. She played that yo-yo game like so many of us. Her weight would never get below 160 pounds. She got to 160 a few times and would be happy for a day or two, but then the weight would creep back onto her small frame.

In her younger years, Deb ranged between 150 to 180 pounds, which at the upper range is a lot for someone who stands at 5'3". When her oldest son was about four, though, she found herself in a terrible place. She couldn't stop eating and felt out of control. She got to a point where she weighed 250 pounds. Imagine that for a moment—5'3" and 250 pounds.

Deb hung around in that range of 225–250 pounds for many years—throughout her son's young years, throughout getting pregnant with her second child. Her kids are seven years apart, so this spanned quite a few years. She was dangerously heavy while pregnant with her second, and there was some fear of losing him. Deb remained in this weight range from about her mid-twenties to about thirty-five years of age.

This was not good. As a nurse, running around heavy didn't send the right kind of message to patients. It was also taxing on her body. Deb eventually realized she has a problem with eating and that she is definitely a binge eater. Fortunately, she doesn't have the purging aspect as that could cause all sorts of other issues. So, she is a binge eater and would eat in excess, then try to start the next day off on the right foot. Deb says she is an all-or-nothing personality, so there is no halfway with her. This is difficult because she is either perfect or terrible.

Deb struggled with this a lot. She would go on bingeing for days and every single morning try to start right, but would immediately get sidetracked. This would result in four or five days of uncontrolled eating, which can put excess weight on a body in a short amount of time. Deb knew she had a problem. Something had to give. She didn't like the person she had become.

Remembering that her father had been a distance runner, Deb started running. She thought it was ridiculous at the time, but she felt that maybe this is what people do to lose weight. Knowing that despite the weight, her heart was healthy, she was healthy, she started the journey slow with the walk-run-walk-run-walk thing. It was a nightmare! Her feet hurt. Everything hurt. But she kept at it. Because she was always the type of person to try and do things, Deb decided she was going to run a marathon.

She recalls that it was crazy out there. Deb was huge and she was running a marathon. Who does that? But she did it and finished in the time that was allowed. She remembers that she couldn't walk to the car afterwards, and joked with her husband that she might need a wheelchair. She actually sat on the ground, then walked a little more, then sat on the ground to get to the car—but she had run a marathon!

This is where Deb's journey towards serious weight loss began. The training and completion of a marathon gave her the push she needed to keep going. With the realization that she could do this, nothing was going to stop her now. So she kept going with the exercise and with running and walking, and pretty soon weight started coming off. Anyone who has ever released weight knows this moment right here is so crucial. Once you see results—you want to see more.

Deb joined Weight Watchers once again and focused this time on trying to learn portion sizes. Shortly after this she found some information on the Paleo diet and tried that, which is still the way she eats today: meats, vegetables, and fruits; real food, not processed. She also eats low glycemic foods and stays away from the so-called "white carbs," such as sugar, white flour, white rice, white bread, potatoes, etc.

Dr. Weil described the Glycemic Index (GI) as a way to categorize carbs by how fast they impact blood sugar levels. The so-called "white-foods" Deb was avoiding are the ones that spike blood sugar quickly. Lower glycemic foods can be found in their natural state, such as wild rice, quinoa, and barley. Essentially, lower GI foods are digested more slowly, thus they are absorbed into the body and metabolized more slowly. This results in a slower rise in blood sugar and in general a lower level than with higher GI foods. Over time, people who eat the Standard American Diet with high GI foods and its accompanying spike in blood sugar may end up with decreased sensitivity to insulin, which can result in things like obesity, high blood pressure, and diabetes, among other things.[107]

As an athlete, Deb did need some carbs, but not things like white bread, crackers, and Cheetos. She adds sweet potatoes to her diet as well as oatmeal. Sugar is a huge trigger for her,

107 Nutrition, Diet, and Q A. 2017. "Confused by the Glycemic Index? – Dr. Weil." Drweil. Com. https://www.drweil.com/diet-nutrition/nutrition/confused-by-the-glycemic-index/ (accessed April 30, 2017).

so Deb tries to avoid it as much as possible. This type of diet is how Deb started eating, and along with measuring or portioning out food, she started to get things under control.

No one is perfect. This was a long journey for Deb because she would periodically slip up and eat too much. Then she wouldn't work out for two days. She would continue to eat and do nothing and kind of go backwards, but not for too long. With her change in diet and the continuation of running, Deb was able to get down close to 200 pounds. This was great compared to 250 and she was feeling good.

At this point Deb decided she wanted to do a triathlon. This was in 2010. She figured she grew up around water and knew how to swim. Not properly, she noted, but she wasn't going to drown. Love this attitude! So she entered and did a little sprint of a triathlon. It took her an hour and fifty minutes to complete. She laughed and said this was crazy for a sprint, but who cares! She completed a triathlon! This particular sprint was a 400-meter swim, a 10-mile bike ride, and a 5k run, which is 3.1 miles. The bike ride alone took Deb an hour and she walked most of the run—but she finished!

This event thrust her into a triathlon kind of lifestyle. Deb always had an underlying strength about her and the ability to do things. This ability and strength enabled her to get her weight down to about 180. And she kept going. She kept doing triathlons. Deb did her first full Ironman in 2012 and she was heavy. It was here that Deb started realizing that she could be good at this, but maybe her weight was holding her back. She was in the "Athena" category, which is for women who weigh over 150 pounds. Athena sounds kind of cool, whereas the heavier category for men is called Clydesdale. That does not sound cool at all, but I digress ...

Triathlon and Ironman races are broken out in categories, such as open/novice/master, with gender, age group, and weight. However, Deb didn't find this very fair. She was 5'3" and 180 pounds and she was competing against women who were 5'10" and 152 pounds. Well, guess who's going to win that race? According to Deb, this has since changed and the Athena category is now for women over 165 pounds.

Deb was starting to want to do well in these races, but she wanted to stop the hurt that always seemed to follow. Because she was so heavy doing it, it was hard on her body. The kicker was that she felt she couldn't tell people she was a triathlete. She felt embarrassed to say these words looking the way she did. She had some fear about hearing the words, "Wow, you don't look like someone who runs triathlons." Deb understands in her head that this is not a good standard to go by. She has seen people much heavier than her, and some much older than her, blow past her in races. Triathlons and marathons have all kinds of body shapes and sizes. None of that matters. These are personal kinds of races, where the only person you are truly competing against is the person you were at your last race.

As a coach, though, Deb wanted to be taken seriously. She wanted to be able to talk about her sport and have people say "of course you're a triathlete." Any health or fitness coach understands this. You want to look the part. You have to walk your talk. How will someone take you seriously as a fitness coach when you are overweight? Even though Deb runs marathons and does triathlons—she's still overweight! Why should anyone listen to her?

This all came to a head about 2.5 years ago, and Deb decided she was going to do another Ironman competition. The one she chose this time, as I'm sure you have guessed by her personality, is one of the most difficult: Ironman Lake Placid. The bike course alone is one of the toughest on the circuit with 7,000 feet of climbing. Deb and her family live in South Florida. Guess what? There are no hills in South Florida. So, climbing on the bike was going to be extremely difficult. Biking was already her weakest discipline.

So Deb, at 180 pounds, had a year to train and prepare for this competition. She knew that to get the results she wanted, she was going to have to do something different. Fortunately, her husband had an answer. He was big into CrossFit at the time and told her if she did strength work, it was going to help her. Prior to this, she always said she never liked strength work and she was never going to walk into that place. Faced with an Ironman, though, Deb sucked it up and started strength training and got serious with her eating. She knew she couldn't fool around and got strict with her diet, and even wrote everything down in a journal.

Writing down everything she ate was key for Deb. She feels that you can't just say "I'm eating clean," because even if you're eating everything clean, you lose track of things and can still overeat. You can't eat three sweet potatoes or an entire chicken and think that's going to be okay. You've got to watch your portions, and tracking your food intake keeps you accountable.

To kick off her strength work in the right way, Deb worked with a coach, who fortunately took her and her goals seriously. This was a very fit guy, and Deb's first impression was that he was going to laugh her right out the door. He didn't and he took her under his wing. He guided her and worked with her privately for a solid year. Once she started the strength work, Deb started building muscle and was able to get to her goal weight: 135 pounds and 12.5% body fat. Impressive!

Today Deb ranges between 135–140 pounds and settled in at 15% body fat, as this is better for her as a distance runner. Her coaches wanted her body weight a bit higher. According to them, when you're running long distance and throwing up on the side of the course, you kind of need something in reserve. We had a good laugh at that.

The Lake Placid Ironman gave Deb her best Ironman time ever. She hit a personal best. It was the fastest time she'd had in any Ironman on any course. She was strong and she felt wonderful. Since that race, Deb continues on the same path. She does CrossFit regularly, still works with her strength coach, trains with a triathlon group, and has her own triathlon coach.

Deb gives credit to journaling her food intake. She tells her clients—just write it down. It doesn't have to be perfect. Even if you screw it up—just write it down. This forces you to remain accountable. On days when your diet is not so great, it's there in black and white. So what. Just do better at your next meal. Write it down.

Water is also crucial to your health, fitness, and weight loss. Most people eat when they really need to hydrate. Try this. Next time you think you're hungry drink a glass of water, and then think about whether you are truly hungry.

There are many components to fitness, according to Deb. There has to be strength work, cardio, and diet. Her ten-year journey to a 115-pound weight loss makes her somewhat of an expert in my book. She says it doesn't matter how long it takes. You can always do something. You can always move forward. If you have weight to lose, I bet you didn't put it on overnight; so you're not going to release it overnight either. It's a journey. And it will probably never be over.

Deb doesn't look at herself and say, "I'm finished." She still attends Weight Watcher meetings. She still journals her food intake. She weighs herself only once per week and tracks how her clothes fit more than the number on the scale. This keeps things real. It's about being aware. Deb also tracks all her workouts. She counsels her clients to just do something. If you can't get a 45-minute walk in, then do 20 minutes. It's worth it. Anything you can do is worth it. It's the little things that add up, and that's how you have success.

Thinking back to her dad, Deb remembered that he had been thin while growing up and then started putting on some weight as a young adult. That's when he turned to running to help manage his weight. This was back in the early 1980s when the running boom first hit. The combination of running and following a strict high-protein diet saw him release the excess weight and be able to maintain it for many years. This was what led her to take up running in the first place. She got inspiration from her dad, who still jogs and follows a high-protein diet to this day. It must be working because at 71 he is healthy and in great shape.

Inspiration:

Her takeaways are this: It's a journey. Embrace the journey. Know it's a process. It takes time. It doesn't happen overnight. You've got to be committed if you seriously want it. You also have to do it for you. You can't do something of this magnitude for someone else, or because of someone else's idea of what you should weigh or how you should look. You can't do this for an event. Or for a man. Or woman. It has to be for you.

Advice:

Deb lives by the quote that opened up this chapter: "the body achieves what the mind believes." I had a different quote for her story, but this one meant so much to her that I changed it. She believes that if you believe you can do something, you will. If you believe you can't, then you are doomed from the start. She counsels her clients to figure out their "why" and write it down. She will push them: Why are you doing this? Why do you want to lose weight? Why do you want to get into shape? When you understand the underlying reason, then you will always have the strength to move forward even in dark times when you are struggling. Your *Why* will help you stay connected to your vision and help you move past the urge to eat the wrong foods or to get up and out the door to exercise on those days when you just want to stay in bed. Your *Why* strengthens your belief that you can do what you set out to do. If you believe you can do something—you will do it.

Contact:

If you like Deb's story and wish to connect with her, or train with her, she can be reached via e-mail at Debbie@3timesfitness.com, on her Facebook group 3 Times Fitness, or at her website: www.3timesfitness.com

Chapter 21

Magdalena: Weight Loss and Family Obligations

A healthy outside starts from the inside.

—*Robert Urich*

Magdalena

Magdalena came to the United States from Poland about fifteen years ago. Poland is in Europe, though there is much controversy about whether it sits in Eastern Europe or Central Europe, and this seems to change over time depending on whom you ask. Nevertheless, Magdalena grew up eating her mother's homemade from-scratch cooking. She was a big believer in "old-fashioned" food preparation and cooking. This meant fresh whole foods; nothing processed. What we call organic today.

Once in the U.S., though, Magdalena's diet changed. As much as she tried to stick to her roots, it's sometimes difficult in this country to eat healthy. It's easy to get caught up in what everyone else is doing. It's easy to become "Americanized" and eat what's available and easy: fast food, packaged foods, processed foods, etc. It's easy to stop at the drive-thru at McDonald's. It's easy to order a pizza on a Friday night after a long week at work.

Then she started dating her now-husband Mark, which typically means dates and dinner out. Things like burgers, pasta, and meatballs found their way into her diet. Over a period of a few years, Magdalena realized she had gained weight. It was a dramatic weight gain of not just a few pounds but about forty to fifty pounds.

It was very difficult for Magdalena to lose this weight. She also began to experience other issues such as high blood pressure and very high sugar levels. She was thirty-five and not terribly concerned about these issues quite yet. But she and Mark were trying to get pregnant and this was proving difficult. Her doctor mentioned that it might be time to look into her diet. Magdalena took offense at this comment. She had begun to change her diet and was trying to do all the right things for a few months now, like cooking at home most of the time. She wasn't sure what to change.

As it turns out they were able to get pregnant, and during this pregnancy, Magdalena lost a lot of weight. Not that she was trying to lose weight—it just happened. After giving birth, the weight came right back on. Magdalena was struggling and decided to do Weight Watchers. She said it was kind of okay, but the idea of counting points was difficult for her. Through this process, though, she did learn about better food choices and proper portion sizes, so that was a win.

She was still on a yo-yo ride, though, as the weight continued to fluctuate and the diet programs she tried expanded. From Jenny Craig, which was unsuccessful for her, to a meal-replacement program, which was okay for a couple of months and then not okay, her weight yo-yoed again. Magdalena was trying whatever new diet was out on the market. She tried them all. You name it—she tried it.

This went on for two years and then she had her second daughter. During this pregnancy, like the first, she lost weight. This is unusual. But again, she couldn't keep it off and regained forty pounds while on maternity leave. Besides all of her weight issues, though, Magdalena was feeling off. She said she was angry, super-sarcastic, obnoxious, bitchy, and yelling all the time. Nothing could make her happy. She hated herself and felt very depressed.

She described it to me this way: "I had a baby and everything was going well, but I felt like I had no joy in life."

Magdalena struggled with this. She didn't know what it was related to and tried talking to someone. Her OB-GYN thought she might have post-partum depression and sent her to a therapist. This made her feel worse—"more lost," as she put it—and she stopped after four sessions. She felt it was going nowhere.

When her youngest daughter was about six months old, Magdalena's husband got very sick. He had developed colitis, which is an inflammatory bowel disease; the more serious version is Crohn's disease. He was not well and there were a few visits to the hospital during this period. Magdalena thought she was going to lose him. He was that sick.[108]

At this point in our conversation, Magdalena mentioned to me that she has this phenomenal cousin in the Midwest who originally trained as an internist but then turned to holistic medicine. She started talking to Magdalena about proper diet, about the need to detox her body, about all the foods she was eating and the fact that they were not exactly as pure as you think they are. She tried to convince Magdalena that changing your diet helps improve your mood and how you feel about yourself. Unfortunately, Magdalena said it went in one ear and right out the other. It was not until her husband got sick and he was put on a ton of medications that she started to pay attention. The medications were helping him physically with his bowel issues, but they were making him sick in other ways. This was the turning point for Magdalena.

Her cousin told her again, "If you just listen to what I'm telling you—if you really listen—I promise you I would be able to take him off this medication." Mark's doctor, on the other hand, was saying that he would never be able to get off these medications; these were long-term medicines and he would be taking them for the rest of his life. No one wants to hear that! Especially when you are in your mid-thirties.

They decided that maybe they should listen to Magdalena's cousin. Right after this, coincidentally two weeks later,

---

108 Wellness, Health, and Mind & Spirit Body. 2017. "Ulcerative Colitis – Dr. Weil's Condition Care Guide." Drweil.Com. https://www.drweil.com/health-wellness/body-mind-spirit/gastrointestinal/ulcerative-colitis/ (accessed February 6, 2017).

Magdalena became very sick and was in the hospital with severe abdominal pains. She said she thought she was having a heart attack. It ended up being her gall bladder. She was told she needed to have her gall bladder removed. She mentioned to her cousin that she didn't want to do the surgery. Her cousin told her the same thing she had been telling her all along: "Why don't you try eating properly? Just try it and see what happens. What do you have to lose?"

Magdalena and Mark slowly started to change their diet, incorporating more greens, greatly reducing gluten, eliminating things like soda and Snapple, buying organic whenever possible, and paying attention to the sources of their food, etc. Her husband also did a vegan detox cleanse and followed a low glycemic diet. Guess what happened? Her husband started getting better, and after six months, he was able to get off all the medications. And ... wait for it. He lost seventy-five pounds.

Wow! Now Magdalena wanted to try and started to listen. Her cousin also sent her some supplements and basically told Magdalena, "Please shut up and just do it. Do it for yourself. You owe it to your kids." After seeing her husband's results, Magdalena was convinced that changing her diet could help. She cancelled her gall bladder surgery and started on a ten-day cleanse. After just those ten days she realized she wasn't waking up in a fog every morning, her mood improved, her skin improved, and she started feeling better about herself, especially when other people started noticing a difference.

She was asked, "What are you doing? What are you on? What changed?" After the ten-day cleanse, which was a kick-start to her total transformation, Magdalena did three back-to-back thirty-day programs, for a total of one hundred days. During that time, she released thirty-eight pounds. This transformation was so much more than physical, though. She had a different outlook on life. She felt so much better about herself and about her body. It changed her mindset. She said it even improved her relationship.

At her annual checkup, her blood work results prompted her doctor to ask her, "What did you change?" She told Magdalena her blood work results were the best she had ever seen in the ten years she had been treating her. "In comparison to where you were a year ago—it's like night and day." She had been thinking about putting Magdalena on blood pressure medication, but now it wasn't necessary.

Before this change, Magdalena felt that everything was crashing. She had turned forty and wondered if this was just a normal part of aging. Now she says, "Life begins at forty!" After all this transformation, with all the weight loss and overall health improvements, with the elimination of medications, with the both of them getting stronger—physically, emotionally, and mentally—Magdalena woke up. Or rather, she broke out of the brain fog that had been muddling her life.

After thirteen years of working in the same place, she changed jobs. Previously she had always been afraid that she wouldn't find anything better. She said she was kind of brainwashed by her boss into staying all those years. She was miserable in that job but felt stuck. After her transformation, once the fog cleared, she thought, *I can do better! I'm going to find something.* And she did just that.

Magdalena now works in a wonderful place with wonderful people in a holistic dental office. She is so much happier and healthier. She also started having more conversations with her cousin, the holistic doctor, and her colleagues. The cousin's sister-in-law is a certified holistic health coach, whom Magdalena spoke with a couple of times over the phone. They became close and Magdalena strongly connected with her and with what she was doing. So much so that she asked her, "How can I learn more about this so I can help people also?"

That's when Magdalena heard about the Health Coach Training Program (HCTP) at the Institute for Integrative Nutrition (IIN). She was so inspired by her cousin and everyone in that practice and by her own transformation that she enrolled in IIN. The combination of her journey and the knowledge she gained through the HCTP gave her the ability and the confidence to help others, even in the dental office where she works.

According to Magdalena, it all comes down to loving yourself and finding time for yourself and your family. Through this process, she learned that her communication style and efforts dramatically improved between her and her husband and their children. There is much more love and support and they listen to each other. Really listen.

Her husband also switched jobs. He had been working for his father and after his transformation, Magdalena told him, "You can do so much better." He was at a new company for about three months when someone higher up took notice of him. He was then pulled up to the parent company, where he is now making more money and is so much happier than he had been working with his father. He feels that he is making a real contribution. He feels needed.

Within a two-year period, they both released weight, got healthier, and changed jobs. Their entire life has transformed—not just their physical bodies. They are happier. Now people are reaching out to them asking about what they did and how they can improve as well. For example, Magdalena was able to help her husband's father, who is seventy-five and was always on the heavy side. She helped him release forty pounds, which was enough to get him off his blood pressure medication. He has a ways to go, but he is already healthier and happier.

Like her father-in-law, Magdalena is a work-in-progress. She is still not where she wants to be, but now she has the strength and the knowledge to do it. She knows there is nothing she can't do. If you believe it—you can achieve it. This transformation also empowered her as a person and as a mother. She said, "I'm just better."

What helped her in this transformation were some products from a particular company which her cousin-doctor has had in her practice for years. Additionally, her cousin's partner is involved in the research. Magdalena believes in this wholeheartedly and says it's not one of those mumbo-jumbo things that she tried before and spent a ton of money on. Her cousin would not put her practice and her license in jeopardy. She wouldn't recommend this to her patients if she didn't truly believe it would help.

Magdalena is so inspired, she wants to tell everyone she meets. She helped a friend who had been recovering from cancer after going through chemotherapy. These products helped her to detoxify and she ended up gaining weight. It's not always about weight loss; for her friend, gaining weight was a good thing, and it was healthy weight and she became stronger. Even her husband, who was once told he would be on crutches for the rest of his life after knee replacement surgery, was transformed with the help of these products. Last summer he ran a Spartan race, which is a kind of running race with obstacles, such as a barbed-wire crawl, spear throw, tire drag, wall jump, and other such things.[109]

As in her husband's case, people hear things from their doctors and believe them to be fact. They think, *this is my fate; this is how it's going to be.* It's disheartening to think about. Magdalena wants people to know this is not true. You can heal yourself within. You can empower yourself. You can change your life.

Two years later both Magdalena and her husband are still healthy and kept the weight off. They are also still a work-in-progress. They are excited to see what future transformations are in store for them. They are eager and enthusiastic to help others transform as well.

Today, Magdalena sees life differently. She feels differently. Guess what? They still eat burgers, they still go to parties, and they still have a glass of wine once in a while. It's not about

---

109 2017. Spartan Race. https://www.spartan.com/en/race/learn-more/obstacle-details (accessed February 12, 2017).

restricting certain things, and it's not about a rigid set of rules to follow. It's about lifestyle. It's about balance. It's about living. One of the basic things they teach at IIN is that wellness is not strictly or solely related to nutrition, though it is a huge factor. It's also about your overall life: your relationships, your career, your spirituality (whatever that means for you), your physical activity, your home environment, your finances, your social life, and things of this nature. If one of those things is out of balance, then you are going to have some stress in your life. Of course, life is never perfect and something will always be shifting. Like Magdalena said, it's a work-in-progress. The main point is to be at peace with yourself.

Inspiration:

Magdalena says her journey through suffering was worth it because of how she feels today. She is so much healthier and stronger. It's not just herself or her self-awareness; it's also that people have seen a change in her and in her husband, and they are now asking what they have done, what they changed. Both Magdalena and her husband Mark have improved their health, their appearance, and their relationship. They are happier and more balanced. So the suffering was worth it to get to where they are today.

Advice:

Magdalena's advice to anyone going through a dark time is to focus on the end goal. See the light at the end of the tunnel.

Literally visualize where you want to be. Visualize what you want to accomplish and what that looks like. See it now, even if you're not there yet. Stay positive. For Magdalena, she wanted better health, she wanted to feel better, she wanted to avoid surgery, and she wanted to be stronger for her kids. That's what she focused on. She visualized herself doing things with her kids that she hadn't been able to do. That kept her going. She had hope and imagination to see where she wanted to eventually be. So, think about your final goal. Visualize yourself in that place. See in your mind where you want to be. Imagine yourself already there. Soon, one day, you will be.

Contact:

If you would like to learn more about Magdalena's transformation or get in touch with her, contact Magdalena Blair, MDT, MS, CHHC at: kaemka@optonline.net, http://clean-burnshape.com/?EnrollerID=87124, http://orendaultimate.com/?EnrollerID=87124, https://mblair.pruvitnow.com/

Chapter 22

Amarjit: Digestive Issues and Stress

Stress is not something that happens to us. It is our response to what happens. And response is something we can choose.

—*Maureen Killoran*

Amarjit

Amarjit's story begins in 2010 when she was living in British Columbia, Canada, with her husband and two children, one boy and one girl. She was also working full time. If you don't know, British Columbia, while extraordinarily beautiful, has a lot of precipitation. The area in which Amarjit lived was lower elevation, so they didn't get much snow, but the rain for days on end could be rather dreary. They lived there for about seven to eight years.

Around this time, Amarjit came to the realization that she wasn't able to digest food very well. She was into homeopathic remedies and tried things like fennel to help with digestion. This didn't work very well, and eventually she realized she was feeling high acidity in her stomach. Whenever she ate she was getting acid reflux. She went to her doctor and he said it's very common, you have a busy life, it's not a big deal, and then asked her about her specific symptoms. Amarjit explained that she felt the food wasn't getting digested, and she felt the acid coming up and she didn't want to eat anymore. The doctor gave her some antacids, which she took for a while.

The symptoms continued, though. Then Amarjit noticed certain foods gave her that gassy, bloated feeling with constipation. She wasn't sure which food caused what, though. Her family has no major health issues, but her father did suffer periodically from constipation, so this wasn't entirely new.

Knowing there was a family history, Amarjit knew she had to do something. She remembered her dad using psyllium husk to help with the constipation, so she did that as well. She would take it at night and feel better in the morning.

But this didn't solve all the issues Amarjit was experiencing, so she went back to the doctor and told him she still didn't feel well. He asked her if she thought stronger antacids would help. Amarjit didn't know but she agreed, so he gave her Nexium to take morning and evening and Gaviscon for heartburn, which she carried in her purse so she would always have it handy.

Then she happened to have a conversation with her pharmacist, who is a strong believer in natural remedies over pharmaceutical drugs when appropriate. He asked Amarjit why she was taking these medications. She told him she didn't want to but she feels better with them. Amarjit knew they weren't curing her. She still felt the same symptoms, but she felt a little better with them than without them.

They spoke about the side effects, and Amarjit reiterated that she didn't want to take these medications and would rather do something natural. The pharmacist agreed. He even joked that as a pharmacist he should just fill her prescription, but he suggested going back to her doctor for further testing because he believed there was something else going on.

So she was trying a lot of home remedies but nothing was working. She is a very strong believer in naturopathic therapies. Amarjit is from India, which is steeped in a rich history of naturopathic medicines. She recalled her mom doing this type of natural stuff when she was growing up, like giving Amarjit turmeric milk at night. Turmeric has been used in healing remedies for over 4,000 years. For example, turmeric milk was used to fight colds as well as boost immunity and help with digestion.[110]

Amarjit's mom would also make teas with lots of herbs and spices. She remembers it tasting good but never thought about why her mom was making these things. Amarjit remembers other things, such as her mom did not like feeding them fruit with food. This I found interesting and had to research. It turns out that the proper way to eat fruit is either by itself or

---

110 "This Happened When I Started Drinking Turmeric Golden Milk Before Bed – David Avocado Wolfe." 2017. David Avocado Wolfe. https://www.davidwolfe.com/turmeric-golden-milk-before-bed (accessed February 6, 2017).

only with other fruit and on an empty stomach. This has to do with the way our bodies break down fruits. Essentially, we use different enzymes to digest fruit than other foods, and if you mix fruit with other foods, the fruit won't digest properly. It will stay in the stomach for too long and either rot or ferment. Fascinating![111]

Amarjit found herself back at her doctor, telling him her symptoms were getting worse. In fact, her acid reflux had gotten to where it wouldn't stop. She was constantly burping and then she would start sweating, so she would go to the bathroom and sit on the toilet for hours. She felt awful physically, but she also felt unclean. Imagine going through life not feeling clean! Amarjit knew something was not right.

This began to happen at Amarjit's place of work as well, which you can imagine is quite inconvenient. It was torturing her. Driving was another problem. Her commute was about thirty minutes one way, and she often had to stop and look for a restroom. She wasn't sure why this was happening or what was going on. She would have gas and stomach pains and acid and was getting very annoyed that the doctor couldn't figure this out.

Finally, Amarjit went to see a gastrointestinal (GI) specialist, who did more blood work as well as allergy testing. He then referred her to get barium testing, which has you drinking barium and then taking a series of X-rays to see what, if anything, is wrong in the digestive tract. The barium is opaque

---

111 "The Major Rule for Eating Fruit." 2017. Mindbodygreen. http://www.mindbodygreen. com/0-4970/The-Major-Rule-for-Eating-Fruit.html (accessed February 6, 2017).

and shows up on X-rays. They were testing for swelling, inflammation, or ulcers. Everything was normal.[112]

Then he sent her for endoscopy, in which a tube with a tiny camera on the tip goes physically down the esophagus. This way the doctor can visually see what the digestive tract looks like. Amarjit was getting frustrated with all the tests and no conclusive results. The doctor explained that he was looking for ulcers in her GI tract. Not liking needles, Amarjit was freaking out. She has a bit of a phobia about needles, and medical professionals often have difficulties finding a viable vein in her arms.

Knowing this, Amarjit spoke up and requested someone who specializes in phlebotomy, which is the person who draws your blood. She told them she might pass out and then they wouldn't be able to do anything. They found a vein for her and proceeded to draw her blood, administer anesthesia, and perform the endoscopy.[113]

The result of this was also normal. However, by this point, Amarjit was fed up and decided to stop taking the Nexium every single day, twice a day. She wondered if it was giving her much more in the way of side effects than it was helping her.

That was how Amarjit spent 2010. She added later that she had been dealing with a stressful family event as well during this year, but at the time she was unable to connect any dots linking her stress-related event to her food issues. This came later.

---

112 "Barium Tests." 2017. Betterhealth.Vic.Gov.Au. https://www.betterhealth.vic.gov.au/health/conditionsandtreatments/barium-tests (accessed February 6, 2017).

113 "Phlebotomy." 2017. Thefreedictionary.Com. http://medical-dictionary.thefreediction-ary.com/phlebotomy (accessed February 6, 2017).

In 2011, she was flying with her family to Mexico for vacation. As you can imagine, they were all excited and had an amazing seven days. Amarjit was very cautious about what she ate while in Mexico and managed to get through the week without too much difficulty. However, when it came time to fly home, trouble started. They were flying from Mexico to Los Angeles and then home to Vancouver.

While waiting for their flight in Mexico, Amarjit had a quesadilla for lunch. Probably not a good idea based on what happened next. After five minutes on the plane, she had a bad reaction to the food she had eaten. She went to the bathroom with severe diarrhea and vomiting. It was so bad that her pulse was falling rapidly due to dehydration. The flight stewards were unable to give her any medication and told her she just had to manage until they reached Los Angeles.

Amarjit's husband was upset. Her children were terrified that something had happened to their mom. They didn't understand what was going on. They had never seen her like this! Her face was pale and colorless. She asked her husband to put some drops of water or juice into her mouth a little bit at a time. There were no doctors on the plane and no one could help her.

The flight crews must have been worried because the pilots pushed the plane a bit and they ended up landing a full thirty minutes earlier than expected. In that time, they had moved Amarjit and her family to business class so that at least she could be a bit more comfortable. Fortunately, the people in those seats moved back to economy to give them some space.

At this point she was not able to talk, she had her eyes shut and her legs up, and she was shivering with cold one moment and then sweating the next. Needless to say—everyone was worried.

Once they landed, Amarjit was rushed to a hospital where they dripped fluids into her. They told her it was most likely food poisoning or something like that and she should follow up with her doctor at home. This whole experience was a bit of a shock to Amarjit, and she came to the realization that indeed something was seriously wrong with her. It was more than simple acid reflux or heartburn. She was determined to get better.

She went back to her doctor and told him the story. He said, "Oh, it was the food you ate in Mexico." She said, "Okay, so what are we going to do now?" They proceeded to test Amarjit for gluten and milk sensitivity. Like all the previous tests, these were also negative.

Back at square one with no answer, Amarjit kept thinking, *so nothing is wrong with me but I have the same problems every single day.* She was experiencing acid reflux every day now at work and at home. She had no relief. And she didn't know why this was happening.

One day someone in her office mentioned the possibility of seeing a naturopath. She had always wanted to, but like many of us, we trust medical doctors. We think they are the ones who know and have answers. She had been believing in them, but she started to lose her faith that they could help. So she went to see a naturopath.

257

The naturopath was not covered by her insurance, but Amarjit was desperate to get better and forged ahead. The doctor suggested a food panel test, which was more comprehensive than anything her previous doctors had done. It was going to cost Amarjit $500 out of pocket, but she didn't care and told the doctor, "Yes, just do it."

This test pointed out that Amarjit was sensitive to seven things: gluten, milk, pineapple, sesame seed, yeast, eggs, and tomato seeds. She also said Amarjit has a leaky gut. Leaky Gut is essentially when you have damage to the intestinal lining due to chronic inflammation and other things. The result is incompletely digested particles seeping through the intestinal walls and into the bloodstream, which leads to more inflammation and can cause autoimmune reactions, gastrointestinal issues, and other disorders.[114]

It was at this point in our interview that Amarjit told me she has a degree in nutrition and has never learned this. Yes, you read that right.

Needless to say, this diagnosis led Amarjit to begin her own research. She started digging into how food is produced in this country, all the damage we are doing, and why so many people are not healthy. She also found that stress was a huge factor in our body's ability to process food. Amarjit came to the conclusion that she needed to reduce or eliminate the stress in her life and somehow get away from the Standard American

114 Wellness, Health, Mind & Spirit Body, and Q A. 2017. "What Is Leaky Gut? – Ask Dr. Weil." Drweil.Com. http://www.drweil.com/health-wellness/body-mind-spirit/gastrointestinal/what-is-leaky-gut/ (accessed February 9, 2017).

Diet (SAD), which is low in fiber and plant-based foods and high in processed foods and animal fats.[115]

We're now into 2013, and for Amarjit to heal herself required a combination of things. First, to get away from the addiction of the Standard American Diet, she followed an almost completely vegan diet. She says it was about 99%, the only exception being ghee or clarified butter (in which the milk solids are cooked off). Becoming almost vegan was not easy given all her food sensitivities, but finally she was able to eliminate the Nexium and Gaviscon from her daily routine. She also started doing yoga, which is wonderful for reducing stress, and she started counseling. This was also difficult for Amarjit, as counseling is not something traditionally done within her culture. She knew it was important, though, as it would help her come to terms with the family-related stress she had been experiencing.

For Amarjit, it was almost a complete lifestyle change. With all the above, she also added exercise into her already full schedule. There was little time for this, but again Amarjit knew it was important to move her body. I say there was little time because another part of her culture requires taking care of elderly relatives and other family members; thus Amarjit's mother-in-law and father-in-law lived with her family. Additionally, her brother-in-law, his wife, and their two teenaged children also lived with Amarjit for about nine months.

---

115 Sears, Dr. 2017. "Standard American Diet (SAD) | Ask Dr. Sears." Ask Dr. Sears | The Trusted Resource for Parents. http://www.askdrsears.com/topics/feeding-eating/family-nutrition/standard-american-diet-sad (accessed April 10, 2017).

Amarjit certainly had her hands full. It was up to her to drop off all four kids at school and handle all the after-school activities, while holding down a full-time job and dealing with all of the above. Add to that all the regular household activities, like cooking for everyone, laundry, cleaning, etc. I'm getting stressed just writing this!

Her job added to her stress as well. Amarjit was a social worker focusing on nutrition. Social work is difficult, and many workers get what is called compassion fatigue from being continually exposed to clients who have suffered. The job of caregivers can be heart-wrenching and emotional, which takes a toll over time. This is a common occurrence and has been compared to posttraumatic stress disorder (PTSD), "except that it applies to those emotionally affected by the trauma of another (usually a client or family member)."[116]

It was at this point in our conversation that Amarjit remembered that the flight scenario she described above while flying home from a family vacation in Mexico happened to her an additional three times. The exact scenario played out three more times. She began to have a fear of flying, as just thinking about what was going to happen almost seemed to trigger it. Sitting in her seat started the process: her palms began to sweat, her husband asked if she was feeling the symptoms, she said yes—and they all left the plane. There were times she would have to argue with the flight attendants to let them off the plane.

116 Harr, C. & Moore, B. (2011). Compassion Fatigue among Social Work Students in Field Placements. *Journal of Teaching in Social Work.* *31*(3), 350–363.

The convincing part of her story was that everyone on the plane would be inconvenienced when she got ill, and no one wanted that! Amarjit laughs about it now. It's funny now—but when it was happening, it was very scary. She recalls a family vacation in 2014 to Florida where this happened. Her kids were so sweet. They told her, "Mommy, it's okay, we don't need to go to Disney World!" What parent wants to hear something like that?! And, of course, the moment she stepped off the plane she was totally fine.

They were rebooked onto a flight, seven hours later, but Amarjit was worried that it would happen again. She called a friend who asked if she wanted to go to a doctor. This wasn't viable in the amount of time they had, so her friend told her to take three glasses of wine and that will relax you. She said, "You just need to relax your mind, go get wine." Amarjit brought her family to a restaurant in the airport and proceeded to get drunk. Not the typical prescription, but in a pinch, it works!

They did eventually make it to Disney World, thanks to some fermented grapes. Afterwards, though, her doctor pre-scribed Ativan, which is for anxiety disorders. Amarjit's family flies a lot, either for vacation or for her husband's work. So it was either take the Ativan or drink three glasses of wine.

For about an entire year, Amarjit worked with her dietary restrictions and became fully vegetarian by choice. Meat was not one of the food groups she had sensitivities to, but she learned so much with all her research about the food industry that she gave it up for good. Fortunately, her husband went along with this; otherwise cooking would have been difficult.

They both stopped eating any kind of living thing. Her husband was entering a more spiritual phase of his life and gave up alcohol as well. This was not a choice for Amarjit, as she wanted to continue to fly and wine helped.

In only about six months, Amarjit says she was a completely different person. She was not ever a heavy woman, but with these changes she managed to release about twenty pounds. That wasn't even a goal for her! She wanted to get better and to stop the acid reflux and heartburn. Her doctor was so impressed that she no longer needed the medications, he wanted to know what Amarjit was doing. He himself took antacids every day, so for him to see Amarjit healthy and not from anything he offered was both fascinating and surprising.

Amarjit learned a lot in this time and thought about all the fighting and struggling inside her mind. She wondered about what was triggering her flight phobia and came to the realization that this was strongly linked to her family stress situation. It was a lightbulb moment. The flight thing was not at all related to food. It was not a reaction to the food she ate. It was from numerous stressful events and situations with her family.

Through counseling, via her own research and her change in lifestyle, Amarjit was able to heal herself. She had experienced so much pain and suffering, but was able to heal herself physically with her new food choices. She also healed herself mentally and spiritually with the help of counseling and soul-searching. For example, she had to learn how to not feel guilty about certain things and some choices she had made; she learned to take responsibility for her choices and not blame anybody else for whatever happened.

Towards the end of 2015, Amarjit had a conversation with her doctor and asked him to redo the food sensitivity panel she had done with the naturopath. She wanted to know if she still had those same sensitivities or if they were merely related to all the stress she had been going through. Her doctor pushed back a little, saying, "You haven't eaten gluten or dairy for about four years now, and if you go for this testing, nothing is going to show on the results." So they came to the conclusion that Amarjit would add these things back into her diet for at least a month and then do the test.

Being cautious and not wanting to dive in too deeply, too fast, Amarjit took it slow. She tried a small piece of bread one day and had no adverse reactions. The next day she ate half a piece of bread; same results. She was surprised that there was no reaction. Happily surprised, but surprised nonetheless. Then one day she ate an entire bagel with cream cheese and was shocked that it was fine. She had no reactions—no acidity and no reflux. Amarjit had repaired her gut and healed her body. She made her immune system so strong that she is now able to digest foods like she had all her life before all this started. As you might imagine, she is a happy camper. She said this was the happiest moment of her life! She remembers the date: November 14, 2015.

This date is when the statement "your brain is in your gut" resonated and solidified for Amarjit. There has been recent research, some of it groundbreaking, on the connection between brain health and the microbiome in our gut. According to David Perlmutter, MD, "The implications of being able to manipulate the health of the blood brain barrier by making changes in the gut bacteria offers up for the first time a powerful therapeutic tool that may have incredibly wide application in brain disorders."[117]

Today, Amarjit and her family live in New York and she can eat anything and everything. She no longer suffers with acidic foods, gluten doesn't bother her, and she has no issues with dairy. She calls herself a healed person. She now has the choice to eat anything. Amarjit is back to where she was about seven years ago, before she had any health issues; before she had so many problems with heartburn, acid reflux, pain, etc. Before all her family-related stress issues made her ill.

Now Amarjit wants to help other people the same way she healed herself. This prompted her to enroll in the Health Coach Training Program at the Institute for Integrative Nutrition. She felt if she could learn more, she could do more and help more people. As mentioned earlier, she has a degree in nutrition, but she never practiced professionally; she was always working in social services. Going through the program at IIN gave her more information on various dietary theories and how to be a health coach, but it was her personal journey that showed her how to heal.

Amarjit recalled a time when she was in Florida and she needed an ambulance. This was at the end of our conversation, and she was remembering that never in her life did she need

---

117 "How Gut Bacteria Protect the Brain." 2017. David Perlmutter, MD. http://www.drperlmutter.com/gut-bacteria-protects-brain/#sthash.Eq3vmvLr.dpuf (accessed February 12, 2017).

an ambulance for herself. So part of this healing journey was that she got to ride in an ambulance. Fun?! She remembers she was going by herself and they were asking her questions, such as "What is your name?" She laughed as she told me her response. She said, "Shut up. I just can't think like this. I need a doctor." The poor EMT was just trying to do his job and get through the procedure. They needed her name. She was in so much pain, though, that she kicked the oxygen tank, which fell on the floor. The EMT backed off and said, "Okay, no more questions." He finally got her into the hospital, and the nurses there piled up fifteen hot blankets on Amarjit's small frame. She was that cold. Fifteen blankets!

These types of stories bring people together. She shares them with friends, family, and sometimes clients to give people a vision of what she went through. This kind of opening up, of being vulnerable, builds trust so that she and her coaching clients have a more meaningful relationship and experience.

Inspiration:

Had she not suffered through her journey, Amarjit would not be who she is today: a healthy, strong woman able to help others on similar journeys. There is no gain without pain. The sad part of Amarjit's story is that she lost her health temporarily and possibly some close family relationships permanently. But on the bright side, she has grown tremendously—mentally, physically, and spiritually.

Advice:

For anyone going through difficult times, Amarjit's advice is to ask for help. Seeking help is what pulled her through her darkest moments. She was dealing with the stress of a broken relationship, alone, in her mind, and it was killing her. Finally she opened up to close friends in the counseling field, who then helped and supported her on a daily basis. Her husband also helped once he realized the depth of the struggle she was dealing with. He stepped up in a huge way to heal the troubling relationship in the family. This one act pulled Amarjit into the light, and she cannot thank him enough for having her back. Looking back with the passing of time and unconscious processing of knowledge, Amarjit can connect all the dots. Our brain is in our gut, and all the food and digestive issues she had been experiencing were all due to the enormous stress she was going through.

Don't wait until it's too late. Seek out help. Talk to someone, anyone, and face your fear.

One of the underlying factors of Amarjit's flight phobia was stress and anxiety. Today, she is phobia free because she fought for this. After healing her gut, she healed her mind with determination, self-love, and support from her husband and friends. She now enjoys traveling with no worries. She enjoys healthy meals of all kinds without stressing over possible reactions. She lives her life to the fullest and loves her husband and children more and more every day. You couldn't ask for a better life than that.

Contact:

The combination of her healing journey and what she learned at IIN is a wonderful foundation for a coaching practice. Amarjit is on a mission to help others who may be going through something similar. She wants people to know that it is possible to heal, that you don't have to rely just on doctors and prescription medications. There is a simple solution in the food we eat. It is possible to heal yourself.

Have you been inspired by Amarjit's story and the brain-gut connection? She is happily helping others through similar journeys and would love to hear from you. Amy Pabbi, MS, INHC, Holistic Nutritionist – www.healinggutnaturally.com

Chapter 23

Sylva: Lack of Energy and Mental Clarity

When diet is wrong medicine is of no use.
When diet is correct medicine is of no need.

—*Ancient Ayurvedic Proverb*

Sylva

My book owes thanks to Sylva because without her, it probably wouldn't exist. Sylva and I met around the time I married my first husband, George. Let's just say it was a long time ago ... Our husbands were best friends. Still are. I've known her husband, Shannon, since he was a student worker in college! Unfortunately, my first marriage ended and even though George and I remained close, over time Sylva and I became somewhat distant. We found ourselves in totally different worlds, where she was married and having babies and I was single again and trying to find myself. We reconnected on

Facebook, though, and kept up with each other's lives through pictures and posts. It was there that I first saw a change in her.

At the time, I was struggling to maintain focus when it came to working on my PhD dissertation. I had successfully completed all my course work and passed my comprehensive examination with flying colors, thus I had "officially attained Doctoral Candidacy status." I was what they call "all but dissertation" (ABD). As exciting as this was, I had lost my passion and was seriously dragging my feet. To the point where I would dread every Sunday night when I had to send an update to the Chair of my dissertation committee on progress I'd made that week. There were only so many times I could write "I've made no progress this week" before it became unsatisfactory and I was kicked out of the program. I was wasting my time and her time and my money and not getting anywhere. Then I saw a post where Sylva wrote something with the words "energy, focus, and mental clarity." That caught my attention! I didn't know what it was that she was doing, but I knew I needed to learn more about it.

Sylva was in her early forties around this time, with two somewhat rambunctious young children; Ava was seven and Alek was three. She was in a terrible funk. Sylva described it as not wanting to be here anymore. And by that she meant living on this planet. She often told her husband that they would be okay without her. He didn't know how to respond. How would anyone respond to their spouse saying they would be better off dead? He didn't understand what she was going through. How could he? For months, Sylva would cry to him at night saying she wasn't well, she wasn't herself, she wasn't a good wife, she wasn't a good mother, she didn't have the energy to live and her family would be fine without her. Sylva was in a very dark place. Emotionally, mentally, and physically. Everything was overwhelming. Living was simply too much for her.

She described it as not feeling well, having no energy, feeling overwhelmed, overstressed, like the walls were closing in on her. She ate what she thought was healthy, but no matter what she tried, she couldn't get herself to feel better. In the past, Sylva tried all different diets and they would start off great, she would release some weight, but eventually it would all find its way back. Now, though, nothing was working. She couldn't lose the weight to even gain it back! Nothing worked.

As a young wife and mom to two children, this was no way to go through life. Her daily life suffered. Her kids, although they didn't know any different, were missing out. Sylva didn't have much energy for anything. She would wake up but wanted to keep sleeping. It was a struggle to get out of bed. She would go through her daily routine because of the kids, and as she put it, you have to do what you have to. But she was literally living on five to six mugs of coffee just to get some energy.

Her children weren't getting her full attention. Sylva wasn't playing with them as much as she wanted to. She was missing so much of their growth as little humans. She had no joy in her kids. At times she would have to ask them to go do their thing and keep quiet. She had a short fuse and even less patience. Fortunately, her children didn't know any better; this is what they were used to and all they'd ever known. They never saw the true spirit of Sylva so they never knew it could be different. Sylva would find herself being a blob on the couch, sitting there catatonic when the kids were in school. Or if the little one was napping, she would take a nap right along with him. She never napped before this! She was doing the bare minimum of what she needed to do for the kids, and couldn't wait for them to go to bed so again she could just be in a catatonic state and a lump on the couch.

Because of all of this, everything piled up and the feeling of overwhelm grew exponentially. She just didn't have the energy to take care of things. That impacted everybody. The entire family. And, of course, it took a toll on her confidence and self-esteem. It took a toll on everything and everyone in her household. Sylva was at a point in her life where she was just done. Mentally, physically, and emotionally ... Done.

Fortunately, a friend introduced her to a nutritional cleansing program that changed her life; the same program Denise and Nicole use. It's a system of products that work together synergistically, all of which are as clean and pure as you can get on this planet. There is a cellular cleanse, a meal replacement shake with active enzymes, and other products made up of vitamins, minerals, botanicals, plant-based adaptogens, and essential nutrients. Sylva, at her wits' end, jumped in with both feet and no hesitation. When you are at the point where you don't want to live anymore, trying one more thing seemed like a no-brainer. She had nothing to lose. And everything to gain.

Within a few days there was a new spark inside of her. Things, feelings were beginning to shift. She had hope that there was a light at the end of the tunnel. Sylva started sleeping more deeply. Her stress seemed to melt away. She worried less about what people thought of her. She had energy. Energy! Weight began to fall off. The world began to look brighter. She was coming out of the darkness. Sylva had belief in life again.

This new spark opened her eyes as to what goes on with food these days and how our food is nutritionally bankrupt. It underscored how important it is to make a concerted effort to eat as close to the earth as possible and to avoid the chemicals, toxins, genetically modified organisms (GMO), pesticides, steroids, hormones, and antibiotics. Additionally, it highlighted for Sylva how we must supplement our nutrition because no matter what we're eating, it is not the same as it was years ago. Our soils today (in the U.S.) have been over-farmed, not rotated as they should have been, and have reduced amounts of the vitamins, trace minerals, and essential nutrients our bodies need to function optimally. In fact, "today's food in the United States is 25 to 50 percent lower in nutrients than it was a half century ago."[118]

After a handful of days into this new nutritional cleansing program, Sylva's energy was sky-high! She was able to manage stress better. She didn't feel so overwhelmed. She slept more deeply and through the night. She had mental clarity and focus that she hadn't experienced in a very long time. After a few weeks, pounds and inches were released. She's been maintaining now for over three years.

The particular cleanse included in this program is chock-full of natural herbs and botanicals that support the body's

---

118 2017. https://bionutrient.org/sites/all/files/docs/2011_Nutrient_Guide.pdf (accessed October 16, 2017).

own filtering system, which includes our liver, kidneys, lungs, spleen, and lymphatic system. When used regularly, the toxins that enter the body every day are prevented from becoming embedded in our soft tissues and cells. Most people don't realize the sheer quantity of toxins and impurities that bombard us on a daily basis. As mentioned earlier, they come from air pollution, car exhaust, water, pesticides, steroids, hormones; even flame-retardants in sofas and carpeting contain harmful chemicals. This never-ending assault has caused our body's natural filters to become so clogged that they cannot keep up with the overload, which results in increased fat. Your body tries to protect itself by encapsulating toxins in fat cells but the longer they remain trapped, the more toxic you become. The importance of a cleanse or supplementation and whole foods is that by ingesting certain nutrients your body is instinctively prompted to repair. A chain reaction is triggered that then decides when, where and how to release toxins so they can't harm other parts of the body. This intricate process of cleansing and re-nourishing is what moves us from sickness to health and that is why it is often called a detox.[119]

Thus, the more conscious we are of supporting our body's natural filters—the more efficient our bodies will work. Most people don't realize how good they are supposed to feel. We are not supposed to feel bloated, have intestinal issues, and experience "aging" aches and pains. That is not natural! It is not just part of the aging process, and Sylva was slowly realizing this.

---

119   2017. http://www.wellnessresources.com/weight/articles/why toxins and waste products impede weight loss - the leptin diet weight (accessed October 16, 2016).

With this new program, Sylva felt as if her body had been reset. If you've ever experienced computer problems, you might understand it this way. When your computer is responding very sluggishly and you reboot it, then everything works faster again. That's how she felt. Rebooted. Like her body was reset to factory standards.

Before starting this program, Sylva's family ate healthy. Any dairy products were all organic and produce was organic as much as possible. It wasn't 100% because at the time, she didn't yet understand the importance of an organic diet. She didn't yet understand the difference between organic and conventional farming and how that manifested in our bodies. She didn't know to look for grass-fed and pasture-raised, etc. But they were eating healthy.

Now Sylva supplements her family's meals with ground turkey, and they eat less red meat and more vegetables. She admits it's still not 100% organic all of the time. Sometimes it's just not available and sometimes you just want to go out for dinner. It's very difficult to be 100% organic. If you can get to 80–90% organic then you're ahead of the game. This is why cleansing is so important, and important to do regularly.

I asked Sylva how long she had felt unwell before beginning this program. She said she always felt it although she never realized it. Like most people, feeling not quite right is something she got used to. Sylva never knew how good she could feel, how good she was supposed to feel, until she started eating clean and supporting her body's natural filters. As she approached forty, she just felt it was a natural part of the aging process, that this is the way we're supposed to feel as we age. Doesn't everybody feel this way? From the age of about twenty, she started experiencing more aches and pains. One day it was her side; another day it was her leg. She thought it was normal to have something hurting. Now she doesn't have that anymore. Now she understands that it's not normal.

Something else Sylva learned with the help of this program is that most Americans are very acidic due to all the packaged and processed chemicalized foods we eat. Disease thrives in an acidic environment. Sylva's body was acidic and had chronic inflammation. This was also diminished with her change in diet. She reflected that she somehow always felt not quite right, but that the older she got the more that ill feeling was pronounced. It increased with each childbirth. But in the months leading up to her starting this program, Sylva felt much, much worse. She wondered if she simply needed to add more exercise, so she hired a trainer who came to the house twice per week. She upped her own workouts as well. This had no effect. Nothing changed. This solidified for Sylva that it's so much more about the food we eat. You can't out-exercise a bad diet. The quote that it's 80% nutrition and 20% exercise hit home for her. She now completely believes this. She lived it!

I never saw Sylva when she was at her darkest. If you saw the woman she is today, you might not believe what came before. Once she changed her diet, her entire lifestyle followed suit. Everything changed when her diet changed. Sylva is whole again—mind, body, and spirit. She got her life back.

Today, Sylva truly enjoys life. She is the vibrant, energetic, caring beautiful woman I knew way back when. It is wonderful to see her full of life and passion. She is so grateful for her nutritional cleansing system that she shares this gift with everyone she knows. And with this gift, Sylva has helped hundreds of people change their lives—both physically and financially.

Sylva's words of wisdom to us all include the fact that sometimes you have to go through something negative and horrible to appreciate the good. Her experience is what motivated her to realize that so many other people must be going through similar dark periods and staying quiet. Let's face it—this is not part of typical conversations. People going through dark times in their life often put on a good face. They are secretly miserable but to the outside world, everything is just fine.

Inspiration:

For Sylva, if she hadn't gone through this dark period, she would never have found the nutritional program that saved her life. She would never have found her true calling. All her life, Sylva knew she wanted to be in a health-related field. Both her parents were doctors, so early on she thought she would end up in the medical field. That didn't feel right, so she thought about dentistry, then physical therapy. Nothing fit. She knew, though, that there was something for her in the health and wellness industry. She would never have found her passion had she not embraced this journey.

She feels that people have to take a deeper look at the negative parts of their life and see what comes out of it. The positive and good and light at the other side can't be appreciated without the balance of the dark and negative.

Advice:

Sylva's advice is to never give up. You may feel like you're in the darkest hole and there's no way out. You might think, well, this is just my life, my path. You might look at others and feel like you're in a dark bubble and everyone else is living in the light. Understand this: you truly can change your circumstance. As horrible as you think it is, as deep as it is, as much as you feel you don't have the energy or the will to even try anymore—sometimes one little thing can make all the difference in the world. You never know what's around the next corner. You never know if or when that one person who's going to be a beacon of light will come into your life. There is always a way. Always.

But if you don't take the entire journey, you won't know this. You won't know there is light at the end. Keep on the path. Just keep going forward. Sylva understands. She knows it can change because she has lived it. She is more credible as a coach today because of her journey through the dark. She is more passionate about helping others today because of her personal journey. Sylva understands the depth of despair people feel because she was there. You can change.

Contact:

If you've been inspired by Sylva and want to reach out or work with her on your own nutritional cleansing, contact her via her personal Facebook page, Sylva Derbarghamian Ortiz, or her community Facebook page, Lifestyle Coaching for Health & Wellness by Sylva. She is also available via e-mail at ortiz.sylva@gmail.com

PART SIX

Changing Your Destiny: Why Genes Don't Have To Have The Final Answer

Chapter 24

Conclusion

I genuinely hope that you have learned something new about the exciting field of epigenetics and that this book has helped open your mind to a new way of thinking. I hope I have shown you that you can have control over healing versus ailing. I sincerely hope that I have given you hope. The amount of material on epigenetics is vast, with over 7,900 (10,000 according to Roazen and Oz) books, articles, academic journals, magazines, newspaper articles, not to mention thousands of alternative health and Google search info results. There is a lot to know in this dynamic, ever-growing field. The good news is that more people are moving towards truly healthy living and not what has been taught to us by the government, including but not limited to the Standard American Diet (SAD).

As I shared, the title *Genetics Isn't Everything* sprouted from my story, from me not getting any of the diseases and conditions that seem to run in my family on both sides of my family tree. I also shared that I am one of those people in an odd situation. Many authors write about their respective experiences and journey through a dilemma, illness, or issue. I've been fortunate enough to remain healthy. I've not been down that road. But as you will learn in my personal story next, I had intuitively started making changes earlier in my life, and I am sure this is part of what has led to my good health.

I hope my goal in writing this book and moving slightly away from the clinical definitions has given new insights. May anyone suffering from a medical illness or watching with fear as hereditary diseases are passed down, know that they don't have to suffer the way their family members have. You can control the destiny of your genes; as a matter of fact, the sum of your actions will create the choice of moving down a path either to ultimate health or chronic illness and early death.

I discussed how genetics most certainly plays a role in who we are and what we are susceptible to. I also want to leave readers with an encouraging feeling and understanding that genetics isn't everything and that you can find a way to en-hance, heal, and help protect the genes you were born with. A little knowledge about genetics and epigenetics can make you stronger, better, and maybe even prevent the illnesses your family has suffered. My point is this: don't give up before you try. Don't live a doomed life going down that path many tra-ditional physicians would lead us. The U.S. is ranked 29th in health and we are supposed to have the best health coverage; seems a bit contradictory to me. I call this sick care, not health care. You can take charge of your health. You can change this.

Bio-individuality is a term I learned recently. It's used a lot these days; makes a lot of sense and has a lot of power. What it means is that we are all unique individuals. Each of us was born with a biome, a biological starting point, and you can't lump an individual with one set of signs or symptoms into a statistic simply because of genetics, a genetic marker, and/or a particular illness such as diabetes. I know people with type 2 diabetes who took charge of their diet early on who now have a perfect A1C and technically don't have to call themselves type 2 diabetics anymore. We need to learn more about this field, research diligently, work on eating right, removing toxins, replacing good bacteria, and alleviating stress—all while finding what our passion is while keeping our body moving with stretching and some exercise and positive thoughts. Sounds like a lot? It's easier than you think once you get started, one small step at a time, and it sure beats the alternative.

This entire book is about empowering you and the people you love to stand up and not live in fear but to take the "genes" by the horns and make them fit you versus living uncomfortably in pain in a body that does not feel good, look good, or function well. Yes, we might have a genetic foundation, a predisposition, but then it is up to us to find a new and healthier path, to build immunity and protection around what we were born with and to live a healthy and happy life. Yes, there are some core diseases that when you are born you will suffer from, and this does fall in the genetic disorders arena. But know this: there is so much more to life that you can become, share, and show that your purpose was never lost on this earth because a gene held you back. You are valued. You are loved and there are people here, like me, to give you help, hope, and strength.

Let me be the first to welcome you to your future "gene-ius!" Now go and live the extraordinary life you were born to lead.

Chapter 25

My Story: Living Your Extraordinary Life

What we do, what we experience,
and how we view the world, along with what
we are exposed to in our environment,
strongly influence the actual outcome of
the genes we inherit.

—Deepak Chopra

Do what you love. Who hasn't heard that at some point in their life? Find something you are passionate about and don't worry about the "making money" part. If you love what you do, it won't feel like a job. If you love what you do the money will follow. More importantly—the happiness will follow! Many times this is easier said than done. Sure, there are those people who know from an early age what they want to be when they grow up, like that five-year-old who wants to be a doctor and never ever wavers from that goal. Then there are others who change with the wind, shifting from one thing to another, but one day they somehow figure it all out.

Life is rarely one extreme or the other, and a majority of people fit into my category: those who are open to whatever possibilities present. I never had a five-year plan. I never had a plan at all. I always knew I would go to college. That was a given. After that—no idea. I didn't know what I wanted to do *in* college—never mind after! My major in college was computer science/mathematics. I chose this because I didn't want to choose the "easiest" major. So, I chose the second easiest. Who does *that*? Although I became pretty good at programming in computer languages, I wasn't too sure I wanted to spend my life doing it. I remember as a junior asking one of my professors about the types of jobs one could get with this degree, hoping he wouldn't say "programmer." Sigh ... he said "programmer." So that's what I did. Thirty years later I'm still with the same organization, in the same department, though I am happy to report that I am doing something completely different. But it's not my purpose. It's not my mission in life. It's getting closer, but it's not what my soul yearns to do.

So, I was never one of those people who knew what they wanted to be when they grew up. In fact, it's only in recent years that I began thinking that I could make a living doing something for which I've always had a passion. You see, from a very young age, I've been interested in health and wellness. Although back then I would not have used those words. I just knew that my family medical history, on both sides of the tree, was not so good. On one side there were all kinds of cancers and Parkinson's and probably stuff I never even knew. The other side had weight issues and anything and everything related to heart disease. This was the legacy I was born into. I knew on some instinctual level that I had to be diligent and somehow learn how to take care of myself. Whatever else would happen in my lifetime—I would be healthy!

As a little kid growing up in the Bronx, I was always active. I remember running around the neighborhood playing all kinds of games with the other kids. Games like tag, paddleball, running bases, stoop ball, and ringolevio (a variation of tag originating from the streets of New York). At one point my friends and I would roller-skate all over the Bronx or ride our bikes to Orchard Beach. We were always outdoors and always in motion. I was part of that generation who left the house early in the morning and came back in time for dinner. We didn't have cell phones; our parents didn't know where we were; we were just out being active and having fun.

That was a different time. The personal computer didn't yet exist. ATMs were still a few years away. We would never have understood sitting in our homes watching a screen or playing an MMPORPG (Massively Multiplayer Online Role-Playing Game). There were no iPads or laptops or mobile phones. There was no such thing as social media—no Facebook, no Twitter, no Instagram, no LinkedIn, no WhatsApp, no Snapchat, and no Pinterest. There was no Internet! We were that generation that went *outside*. We ran around and played. We interacted with other children face-to-face—in "real life," in "real time."

When I was a high school sophomore, I joined the track team and began a love-hate relationship with running which lasted just about thirty years. The beginnings of arthritis in the ball of my right foot put that to an end. I stopped running and it stopped hurting. At first I would still feel it once in a while like on rainy days and after wearing heels, but as my diet got cleaner and cleaner even that seemed to go away. Even in college I was active in sports, and afterwards always had some form of exercise routine, and still do to this day.

My favorite form of exercise today is using my Incline Trainer.[120] It's like a treadmill, but has a shorter tread and goes up to a 40% incline, so you burn more calories in a shorter amount of time than a traditional treadmill. That's my go-to workout. I begin walking at 3 miles per hour at a 20% incline and raise the incline every ten minutes or so. I also vary how I do it. In other words, sometimes I hold onto the bars so I'm also getting a slight upper-body workout; sometimes I work my core by not holding on. I would love to tell you that I also do yoga. Alas, I would be lying. Years ago, I did yoga three to four times per week and was in the best condition of my life. I keep telling myself that I need to get back into yoga, but to date that hasn't happened yet. I do stay flexible by stretching three times each week, and I have an eighteen-pound bar that I use a few times per week to work my muscles.

Physical activity was always a given. It was always part of my life. Then there were the quirky things I did that I didn't fully comprehend at the time. Little odd things come to mind, like never wanting to use the microwave to heat things up. There was just something that bothered me about using a microwave. It didn't seem natural. While writing this, I dug a little

---

120 Trainers, Incline, X9i Trainer, X22i Trainer, and X11i Trainer. 2017. "Incline Trainers Treadmills | Nordictrack.Com." Nordictrack.Com. https://www.nordictrack.com/incline-trainers (accessed April 10, 2017).

deeper and found out that using a microwave actually changes the chemical structure of what you're heating up. According to an article on Dr. Mercola's website, "Microwaving distorts and deforms the molecules of whatever food or other substance you subject to it."[121] It takes away some of the nutrients of the food and makes others carcinogenic. No thank you.

I also avoided Styrofoam and never wanted to store food in plastic containers. I specifically bought glass containers to store leftover food so I could avoid using plastic. I didn't know why, I just had some intuition that glass was better. I've since learned that some of the chemicals in plastic containers, plates, and utensils can leach into the food you are eating. This can lead to insulin resistance, which can lead to inflammation, which can lead to serious health issues. As a start there are now BPA-free plastics (bisphenol A)[122] you can find, but I'm not taking any chances.[123]

Another thing I just thought of: whenever I bring clothes home from the dry cleaners, which is rare, I immediately take the clothes out of the plastic bags and hang them on the shower rod or somewhere else where they can air out for a few days. Then I wait at least a week before I'll put anything dry-cleaned back on my body. Apparently, there is a chemical used by most dry cleaners that has been known to cause

---

121 "The Hidden Hazards of Microwave Cooking." 2017. Mercola.Com. http://articles.mercola.com/sites/articles/archive/2010/05/18/microwave-hazards.aspx (accessed April 10, 2017).

122 "What Is BPA? Should I Be Worried About It? – Mayo Clinic." 2017. Mayo Clinic. http://www.mayoclinic.org/healthy-lifestyle/nutrition-and-healthy-eating/expert-answers/bpa/faq-20058331 (accessed 4.11.2017).

123 Wellness, Health, Balanced Living, Healthy Living, and Q A. 2017. "Are Plastic Containers Unhealthy? – Drweil.Com." Drweil.Com. https://www.drweil.com/health-wellness/balanced-living/healthy-living/are-plastic-containers-unhealthy (accessed April 10, 2017).

cancer in animals.[124] Not for me, thank you. I'll be looking for a green or organic dry cleaner.

I've always had an aversion to taking any over-the-counter medication, and to this day my husband has to yell at me to take an ibuprofen if I have a headache. I'd rather drink more water and perhaps eat something to see if it dissipates. I've even avoided prescribed medication when I could. For example, I never took any birth control. Never. Of course, I would take antibiotics when needed, but if I knew back then what I know today, I might have fought that a little harder.

Thankfully these weird habits I had kept me healthy. At least I think they did. I mean, I am in excellent health, so they must have had some input. Right? Then I started slowly changing my diet by incorporating organic food. I'm not entirely sure what precipitated this, though I imagine I started hearing more about organic food in the news. In 1990, "Congress passed the Organic Foods Production Act (OFPA)," which may be where it all began for me. Earlier, in the 1970s, there was "increased environmental awareness and consumer demand,"[125] though I would have been too young to be aware of it back then. Around this same time, I started eliminating most processed foods; I stopped drinking soda and began reading food labels much more carefully. All of these habits built upon each other and increased over the years.

---

124 Wellness, Health, Balanced Living, Healthy Living, and Q A. 2017. "Do You Green Dry Clean? – Drweil.Com." Drweil.Com. https://www.drweil.com/health-wellness/balanced-living/healthy-living/do-you-green-dry-clean/ (accessed April 10, 2017).

125 Nationwide, SARE. 2017. "History of Organic Farming in the United States." Sare.Org. http://www.sare.org/Learning-Center/Bulletins/Transitioning-to-Organic-Production/Text-Version/History-of-Organic-Farming-in-the-United-States (accessed April 10, 2017).

Yet, even with all of this, I found myself exhausted. Fast-forward to 2014. I thought I was eating clean, but I was still exhausted. I would come home from my full-time job every day and feel exhausted. There is no other word for it. I was physically, mentally, emotionally, and even spiritually—exhausted. I got home, changed out of my work clothes, and then sat on the couch and mindlessly watched the television. My husband would cook for us most nights, and we would eat on the couch watching the television. At the time I was writing my PhD dissertation and I couldn't even think about getting up from that couch, walking over to my computer, and doing more work. It just wasn't happening. I had lost something. My passion was gone. I kept thinking that if I had my energy back, I would find my passion again.

It was right around this time that I started noticing Sylva (see chapter 23) posting things on Facebook about getting her life back, feeling alive again, releasing stubborn baby weight, etc. I watched this for a few months until one day she wrote the words "energy, focus and mental clarity." Wow! That struck a nerve. I didn't know what it was that she was doing, but I knew I needed to find out more.

We spoke on the phone that very day and I ordered one of the nutritional cleansing systems. I received my box on a Tuesday evening and started the very next day. The program is all about nutrition and putting the best-quality food into your body that you can with enzymes to support the digestive process.

Day five into this program I had a lightbulb moment. It was late in the afternoon on a Monday and I was in my office at work. I remember sitting back in my chair around 3:30 pm and thinking, *Wow! That was the most productive day I've had in more months than I care to admit.* I don't remember what I was working on. I just remember all the information I needed simply flowed into my brain. I was in the zone or in a state of flow or Zen or whatever you want to call it. It was a magical moment that I will never forget. The focus and mental clarity I had on that day was unparalleled. I had never experienced that before in my life. Not that I could remember, anyway.

With this newfound energy, focus, and mental clarity, I knew I needed to become even more resolute about my diet and that of my husband. We went from sometimes organic to about 80% organic. The only beef we brought home was grass-fed. Fish was wild-caught. GMOs were not allowed. We started making more vegetables and salads with our meals. We switched to extra-virgin olive oil instead of vegetable oil. We learned about superfoods and started eating avocados every day; added more blueberries, almonds, and sweet potatoes into our routine. I was already adding cinnamon to my coffee every morning, so that was a plus! And instead of cream, I blend my coffee with coconut oil. Snacks were nuts instead of cookies. Corn chips were eliminated in favor of bean chips. We very carefully read labels. Even spices and coffee became organic.

Right around this time, I noticed many advertisements on social media about the Health Coach Training Program at the Institute for Integrative Nutrition (IIN). It's scary sometimes what pops up on your feed—all based upon what you post. Apparently, I had been posting more about nutrition, health, weight loss, etc., and somehow Facebook knew this and thought I would be interested in ads around health, nutrition, etc. Well—Facebook was right. One day I clicked on an ad for IIN and took a sample class. Then I began the yearlong program that propelled me into a new trajectory.

That yearlong course gave me much-needed information about nutrition, dietary theories, and food. It also gave me the necessary tools to become a health coach and the confidence to know that I can truly help people. That yearlong course led me to a follow-on course about writing your dream book—this book. This is why I wrote that this book would probably never have happened were it not for Sylva. The dots all link back to her.

Self-care also became much more important to me. I was always one for getting monthly massages, and that hasn't stopped. What I learned through the years, though, is that self-care, self-love, and self-compassion are crucial for our overall wellness. But this can't be forced. It has to be a natural extension of who you are. Self-care doesn't mean go take a yoga or Pilates class if that's not something that interests you. It doesn't mean go get a massage if that's out of your budget. Self-care can be as simple as taking a bath. Or a walk. There is no prescription for self-care. There is no right or wrong way to do it. It's time to yourself, for yourself, in whatever way works for you and your lifestyle. It's that simple.

I used to dabble with meditation, and if you know anything about meditation, you know it doesn't work that way. The more consistent you are, the better it works. So, I bought a Muse headphone device thingy. Yes, that's the technical term. Okay, it's actually called MUSE, the brain sensing headband, and it is very cool. It essentially senses your brain waves and knows when you are in a calm, neutral, or active state. It charts this for each session that you save, so you can see graphs and manage your progress over time. Like I said, very cool, if you are a visual person like me. The point, though, is that my meditation practice has become much more consistent. I meditate for twenty minutes most days, and I can see that my brain is more and more in a calm state rather than an active state. Meditation has been shown to improve physical health and mental health. It lowers stress and it can help with depression and anxiety.[126]

Oh, in case you're wondering, I officially withdrew from my PhD program. Even though my dissertation was about compassion, it was focused on compassion in the workplace. I realized that my workplace was not where I wanted it to be. I realized that my passion was no longer in organizational leadership and that it's more aligned with writing books and working closely with people, especially one-on-one in my coaching practice. I have found my calling.

I'm on a mission to spread hope. My passion is to help people understand that genetics isn't everything. Just because you have certain family traits and genes or certain diseases seem to run in your family, there is no guarantee that you will get the same diseases or conditions your parents or grandparents had. If you've gotten this far in my

126 "Meditation Benefits: An Interview with Susan Piver – Drweil.Com." 2017. Drweil.Com. https://www.drweil.com/health-wellness/balanced-living/meditation-inspiration/an-interview-with-susan-piver (accessed April 10, 2017).

book, then you've read all the stories about people who have changed their health and thus their lives with nutrition and self-care. A happy and healthy life, while not guaranteed to everyone, *is within reach*. You *can* change your health with nutrition and self-compassion. You can take your life back.

There is no magic pill, though. If you choose to embark on this journey, you may have a huge uphill battle on your hands. You may have to go against advice of those you hold dear. You may have to stand alone. This will take a lot of effort and dedication and time. In the end, however, it is totally worth it.

I wanted to end this book with my story because it's very different from what came before. Unlike the other stories, I had no health issues to overcome. I didn't reverse or alleviate some disease. I did not change my health with nutrition, at least not in an obvious way. I won't go as far as to say that I prevented certain diseases from manifesting in my body. I do, however, absolutely believe that I kept myself healthy. I am in perfect health. I know that I've been able to achieve this with my life choices. Sure, I have issues with my weight, and I've struggled with self-esteem and confidence because of my weight since I was about fourteen. I'm also pre-menopausal. I can't avoid that. But I've come to accept my body. It's taken me about 50 years, but I've learned to *love* my body. I accept my so-called imperfections because most of them are someone else's idea of what perfection should be. I am healthy. Seriously. Healthy. That is more important to me than how I look to others.

I have lived on planet Earth for 52 years. And, I have no

health issues. None. I don't take any prescription medications. Zero. I have no allergies. I am in perfect health. I also live an extraordinary life! I travel. A lot. I write. I work. I eat healthy foods. Really, really good healthy foods. I exercise. I drink water. I drink wine. I ski in the winter. I also camp in the winter. I love to hike. I love to watch movies. I love trying new restaurants. I love getting massages. My life is very full and very happy.

When I say I live an extraordinary life, though—that's by my definition. Your definition may be very different. I want you to think about all that I shared and then actively take a few recommendations or stories to heart. Care enough about yourself to move towards optimal health. My goal in life is to help you find *your* extraordinary. As I said in the introduction and as is confirmed by these stories, it can be easier and faster than you ever imagined when you build reinforcements for those genes. Who knows, your side effect might just be fitting into your jeans better—and who wouldn't love that?

Be healthy, play hard, spread love and knowledge, and now, go have fun!

Bibliography

"5 Natural Remedies for Fibromyalgia – Draxe. Com." 2017. *Dr. Axe.* https://draxe.com/ natural-remedies-for-fibromyalgia/

"9 Charts That Show the Standard American Diet." 2017. *Dr. Axe.* https://draxe.com/charts-american-diet

"10 Reasons Why You Should Eat Local." 2017. *Ecowatch.* http://www.ecowatch.com/10-reasons-why-you-should-eat-local-1882029859.html

2017. https://apstudent.collegeboard.org/exploreap/ the-rewards

2017. http://articles.mercola.com/ sites/ articles/archive/2017/04/13/ depression-leading-cause-of-illness-disability-worldwide

2017. http://www.askdrsears.com/topics/feeding-eating/ family-nutrition/standard-american-diet-sad

2017. https://bionutrient.org/sites/all/files/docs/2011_ Nutrient_Guide.pdf

2017. http://drhyman.com/blog/2016/05/12/8-tips-to-ease-detox-discomfort/ retrieved

2017. http://www.greenfacts.org/en/endocrine-disruptors/endocrine-disruptors.htm

2017. IRONMAN.Com. http://www.ironman.com/

2017. *Isitbadforyou.Com.* https://www.isitbadforyou.com/questions/is-carrageenan-bad-for-you

2017. http://www.lupus.org/answers/entry/is-lupus-hereditary

2017. http://www.lupus.org/answers/entry/where-did-the-name-lupus-come

2017. http://www.mayoclinic.org/diseases-conditions/migraine-headache/home/ovc-20202432

2017. http://www.mg217.com/your-psoriasis/statistics-about-psoriasis

2017. http://www.modernmom.com/2c3cf2b0-051f-11e2-9d62-404062497d7e.htm

2017. http://www.nature.com/jhg/journal/v60/n11/full/jhg201594a.html

2017. https://www.psoriasis.org/about-psoriasis/treatments/phototherapy

2017. https://www.spartan.com/en/race/learn-more/obstacle-details

2017. http://www.sustainabletable.org/248/
sustainable-livestock-husbandry

2017. https://www.theatlantic.com/health/archive/2016/12/
why-are-so-many-americans-dying-young/510455/

2017. http://www.webmd.com/mental-
health/eating-disorders/news/20001117/
orthorexia-good-diets-gone-bad

2017. https://weillcornell.org/rheumatology

2017. http://www.wellnessresources.com/weight/articles/
why-toxins-and-waste-products-impede-weight-loss-the-
leptin-diet-weight

"A Sleepless Night Can Wreck Your DNA." *Daily Mail*
(London), July 23, 2015.

Anderson, E. N. *Everyone Eats: Understanding Food and
Culture*. 2nd ed. New York: New York University Press,
2014.

Andreasen, Nancy C. *Brave New Brain: Conquering Mental
Illness in the Era of the Genome*. New York: Oxford
University Press, 2003.

"Are Migraines Hereditary?" 2017. *Migrainehelper.Com.*
http://www.migrainehelper.com/migraine-occurrence-
in-women-and-families.shtml

Arrison, Sonia. *100 Plus: How the Coming Age of
Longevity Will Change Everything, from Careers and
Relationships to Family and Faith*. New York: Basic
Books, 2011.

Articles, Latest, Ask FAQs, Mark's Minutes, TV Media, and MD Mark Hyman. 2017. "About Functional Medicine – Dr. Mark Hyman." *Dr. Mark Hyman.* http://drhyman.com/about-2/about-functional-medicine/

Avise, John C. *The Hope, Hype & Reality of Genetic Engineering: Remarkable Stories from Agriculture, Industry, Medicine, and the Environment.* New York: Oxford University Press, 2004.

"BBC – GCSE Bitesize: The Discovery Of DNA." 2017. *Bbc.Co.Uk.* http://www.bbc.co.uk/schools/gcsebitesize/science/add_edexcel/cells/dnarev3.shtml

"Barium Tests." 2017. Betterhealth.Vic.Gov.Au. https://www.betterhealth.vic.gov.au/health/conditionsandtreatments/barium-tests

Barnes, Barry, and John Dupré. *Genomes and What to Make of Them.* Chicago: University of Chicago Press, 2008.

Beal, Tom. "Thanks to Complex Field of Epigenetics, It's Now Clear 'DNA Is Not Your Destiny.'" *AZ Daily Star*, February 24, 2013.

Beal, Tom. "We Travel the Road to 'Mastery of Our Biological Destiny.'" *AZ Daily Star*, January 27, 2013.

"Birth Defect Statistics." 2017. *The Physicians Committee.* http://www.pcrm.org/research/resch/reschethics/birth-defect-statistics

Boey, Bernard. 2017. "Maternal-Fetal Medicine | Obstetrics and Gynecology | Weill Cornell Medical College." Cornellobgyn.Org. http://www.cornellobgyn.org/clinical-services/maternal-fetal-medicine.html

Brigham, Kenneth, and Michael M. E. Johns. Predictive Health: How We Can Reinvent Medicine to Extend Our Best Years. New York: Basic Books, 2012.

"Cancer Statistics." 2017. *National Cancer Institute.* https://www.cancer.gov/about-cancer/understanding/statistics

Caplan, Arthur. "Old Rule against Genetically Altering Heritable Traits Is History." *Examiner* (Washington, D.C.), December 5, 2015.

Caporale, Lynn Helena, ed. *The Implicit Genome.* New York: Oxford University Press, 2006.

"Chronic Migraine by the Numbers." 2017. *My Chronic Migraine.* https://www.mychronicmigraine.com/living-with-chronic-migraine?cid=sem_goo_43700007344044820

Clark, William R. *The New Healers: The Promise and Problems of Molecular Medicine in the Twenty-First Century.* New York: Oxford University Press, 1997.

"Clean Your Body's Drains: 10 Ways to Detoxify Your Lymphatic System." 2017. *Healthy and Natural World.* http://www.healthyandnaturalworld.com/natural-ways-to-cleanse-your-lymphatic-system/

Cold, Flu & Cough, Eye Health, Heart Disease, Pain Management, Sexual Conditions, Skin Problems, and Sleep Disorders et al. 2017. "What Is Acid Reflux Disease?" Webmd. http://www.webmd.com/heartburn-gerd/guide/what-is-acid-reflux-disease?page=3

Coll, Cynthia Garcia, Elaine L. Bearer, and Richard M. Lerner, eds. *Nature and Nurture: The Complex Interplay of Genetic and Environmental Influences on Human Behavior and Development.* Mahwah, NJ: Lawrence Erlbaum Associates, 2004.

"Conditions That May Be More Than Just Skin Deep." *Hindustan Times* (New Delhi, India), July 13, 2015.

Corwin, Tom. "Cancer Center Tries to Make a Reputation in Epigenetics; It's Finding How DNA Can Be Changed without Changing the Genetic Code." *The Florida Times Union*, August 22, 2006.

"Course Overview: Your Infinite Life." 2017. Yourinfinitelifeonline.Com. https://www.yourinfinitelife-online.com/courses.php

"Cracking the Code Advances in Genetic Testing Allow for More Personalized Medical Treatments." *Daily News* (Los Angeles, CA), June 28, 2012.

"Crossfit: Forging Elite Fitness: Sunday 170514." 2017. Crossfit.Com. http://www.crossfit.com

"Detailed Findings." 2017. *EWG.* http://www.ewg.org/research/body-burden-pollution-newborns/detailed-findings

"Don't Blame Your Genes: Science Can Help Change Them." *Daily Mail* (London), March 30, 2010.

Driver, Catherine Burt MD. 2017. "Fibromyalgia Symptoms, Treatment, Causes – Is Fibromyalgia Hereditary? – Medicinenet." *Medicinenet.* http://www.medicinenet.com/fibromyalgia_facts/page2.htm

"Epigenetics: Fundamentals – What Is Epigenetics?" 2017. *What Is Epigenetics?* http://www.whatisepigenetics.com/fundamentals/

"Exercise to Optimize Your Health – Mercola.Com." 2017. *Fitness.Mercola.Com.* http://fitness.mercola.com/sites/fitness/exercises.aspx

"Faststats." 2017. *Cdc.Gov.* https://www.cdc.gov/nchs/fastats/leading-causes-of-death.htm

Feinberg, Arthur N. "Dermatology: Intellectual and Developmental Disabilities." *International Journal of Child Health and Human Development* 8, no. 3 (2015): 365+.

Fossel, Michael B. *Cells, Aging, and Human Disease.* New York: Oxford University Press, 2004.

Fraser, Gary E. *Diet, Life Expectancy, and Chronic Disease: Studies of Seventh-Day Adventists and Other Vegetarians.* New York: Oxford University Press, 2003.

"Free Calorie Counter, Diet & Exercise Journal | Myfitnesspal.Com." 2017. Myfitnesspal.Com. http://www.myfitnesspal.com/

Genetics. 2017. "Can Changes in Mitochondrial DNA Affect Health and Development?" *Genetics Home Reference.* https://ghr.nlm.nih.gov/primer/mutationsanddisorders/mitochondrialconditions

Genetics. 2017. "How Many Chromosomes Do People Have?" *Genetics Home Reference.* https://ghr.nlm.nih.gov/primer/basics/howmanychromosomes

Genetics. 2017. "What Is a Gene Mutation and How Do Mutations Occur?" *Genetics Home Reference.* https://ghr.nlm.nih.gov/primer/mutationsanddisorders/genemutation

Genetics. 2017. "What Is a Gene?" *Genetics Home Reference.* https://ghr.nlm.nih.gov/primer/basics/gene

"Genetics of Migraine Headaches." 2017. *En.Wikipedia.Org.* https://en.wikipedia.org/wiki/Genetics_of_migraine_headaches

Gluckman, Peter, and Mark Hanson. *Mismatch: Why Our World No Longer Fits Our Bodies.* New York: Oxford University Press, 2006.

Goldschmidt, Richard B. *Understanding Heredity: An Introduction to Genetics.* New York: Wiley, 1952.

Happe, Kelly E. *The Material Gene: Gender, Race, and Heredity after the Human Genome Project.* New York: New York University Press, 2013.

"Health Protocols | Life Extension." 2017. *Lifeextension. Com.* http://www.lifeextension.com/Protocols/Metabolic-Health/Thyroid-Regulation/Page-les

"History of Fibromyalgia." 2017. Healthcentral.Com. http://www.healthcentral.com/chronic-pain/fibromyal-gia-287647-5.html

"Home – Maddy Moon." 2017. Maddy Moon. http://maddy-moon.com/

"How Gut Bacteria Protect the Brain." 2017. David Perlmutter, MD. http://www.drperlmutter.com/gut-bac-teria-protects-brain/#sthash.Eq3vmvLr.dpuf

"How to Get Rid of Vertigo – Dr. Axe." 2017. Dr. Axe. https://draxe.com/how-to-get-rid-of-vertigo

"Hypothyroidism Diet + Natural Treatment – Dr. Axe." 2017. *Dr. Axe.* https://draxe.com/hypothyroidism-diet-natural-treatment/

"Inflammation and Its Diseases." *Nutrition Health Review*, January 1, 2013, 2+.

"Is Soy Bad for You? – Dr. Axe." 2017. Dr. Axe. https://draxe.com/is-soy-bad-for-you/

"Is Your Body Begging You to Go Macrobiotic?" 2017. *Dr. Axe.* https://draxe.com/macrobiotic-diet/

Jablonka, Eva, and Marion J. Lamb. *Epigenetic Inheritance and Evolution: The Lamarckian Dimension.* Oxford: Oxford University Press, 1995.

Jacoby, David B., and Robert M. Youngson, eds. *Encyclopedia of Family Health.* 3rd ed. Vol. 7. New York: Marshall Cavendish, 2005.

"Joshua Rosenthal's Bio-Individuality Is Scientifically Proven." 2017. *Institute for Integrative Nutrition.* http://www.integrativenutrition.com/blog/2015/07/joshua-rosenthal-s-bio-individuality-is-scientifically-proven

Karlsson, Jon L. *Genetics of Human Mentality.* New York: Praeger Publishers, 1991.

Kasper, Siegfried, and George N. Papadimitriou, eds. *Schizophrenia.* 2nd ed. Medical Psychiatry. New York: Informa Healthcare, 2009.

Khazan, Olga. 2017. "Why Americans Die Younger Than Europeans." *The Atlantic.* https://www.theatlantic.com/health/archive/2016/12/why-are-so-many-americans-dying-young/510455/

Lawrence, Glen D. *The Fats of Life: Essential Fatty Acids in Health and Disease.* New Brunswick, NJ: Rutgers University Press, 2010.

Lee, Thomas F. *The Human Genome Project: Cracking the Genetic Code of Life.* New York: Plenum Press, 1991.

"Lifestyle Wins over Genetics; Our Healthy Choices Have Huge Impact." *The Observer* (Gladstone, Australia), October 6, 2016.

McCabe, Linda L., and Edward R. B. McCabe. *DNA: Promise and Peril.* Berkeley, CA: University of California Press, 2008.

McElheny, Victor K. *Drawing the Map of Life: Inside the Human Genome Project.* New York: Basic Books, 2012.

"Meditation Benefits: An Interview with Susan Piver
– Drweil.Com." 2017. Drweil.Com. https://www.
drweil.com/health-wellness/balanced-living/
meditation-inspiration/an-interview-with-susan-piver

"MUSE ™ | Meditation Made Easy." 2017. Muse: The Brain
Sensing Headband. http://www.choosemuse.com/

Myers, Amy. MD, 2017. "9 Foods to Ditch If
You Have Candida – Amy Myers, MD." *Amy
Myers, MD*. http://www.amymyersmd.
com/2016/07/9-foods-to-avoid-if-you-have-candida/

Nationwide, SARE. 2017. "History of Organic
Farming in the United States." Sare.Org. http://
www.sare.org/Learning-Center/Bulletins/
Transitioning-to-Organic-Production/Text-Version/
History-of-Organic-Farming-in-the-United-States

Neff, Kristin, What Self-Compassion?, What Self-
Compassion?, What Not, Tips Practice, Videos Self-
Compassion, and MSC Intensives et al. 2017. "Definition
and Three Elements of Self-Compassion | Kristin
Neff." *Self-Compassion*. http://self-compassion.org/
the-three-elements-of-self-compassion-2/

"No-Amylose Diet | Surviving Mold Illness." 2017.
Survivingmoldillness.Com. http://www.survivingmoldi-
llness.com/no-amylose-diet.

Norman, James MD, FACE. 2017. "Hypothyroidism:
Overview, Causes, and Symptoms." *Endocrineweb*.
http://www.endocrineweb.com/conditions/thyroid/
hypothyroidism-too-little-thyroid-hormone

Nutrition, Diet, Anti-Inflammatory Pyramid, and Dr. Pyramid. 2017. "Dr. Weil's Anti-Inflammatory Food Pyramid | Anti-Inflammatory Foods." *Drweil.Com.* http://www.drweil.com/diet-nutrition/anti-inflammatory-diet-pyramid/dr-weils-anti-inflammatory-food-pyramid

Nutrition, Diet, Food Safety, and Q A. 2017. "Carrageenan Dangers – Carrageenan Safety | Dr. Weil." *Drweil.Com.* http://www.drweil.com/diet-nutrition/food-safety/is-carrageenan-safe/

Nutrition, Diet, and Q A. 2017. "Confused by the Glycemic Index? – Dr. Weil." Drweil.Com. https://www.drweil.com/diet-nutrition/nutrition/confused-by-the-glycemic-index/

"Orthorexia." 2017. *National Eating Disorders Association.* https://www.nationaleatingdisorders.org/learn/by-eating-disorder/other/orthorexia

Pauwels, Eleonore. "Our Genes, Their Secrets." *International Herald Tribune,* June 2, 2013.

Pearson, Thomas. "Inflammation and Its Diseases." *Nutrition Health Review,* Spring 2012, 2+.

"Phlebotomy." 2017. Thefreedictionary.Com. http://medical-dictionary.thefreedictionary.com/phlebotomy

"Plaquenil Uses, Dosage & Side Effects – Drugs.Com." 2017. *Drugs.Com.* https://www.drugs.com/plaquenil.html

"Radiate My Thyroid? What?! No Freakin' Way! – Andrea Beaman." 2017. *Andrea Beaman*. http://andreabeaman. com/radiate-my-thyroid-what-no-freakin-way/

Ramos, Paula S., Andrew M. Shedlock, and Carl D. Langefeld. 2017. "Genetics of Autoimmune Diseases: Insights from Population Genetics."

Roizen, Michael MD. "You're Only as Old as the Choices You Make." *Telegraph – Herald* (Dubuque), March 16, 2016.

Roizen, Michael MD, and Mehmet Oz, MD. "6 Ways to Switch on Your Healthy, Happy Genes." *AZ Daily Star*, February 16, 2015.

"Role of the Thyroid | Life Extension." 2017. *Lifeextension. Com*. http://www.lifeextension.com/Protocols/ Metabolic-Health/Thyroid-Regulation/Page-02

Sargis, Robert M., MD, PhD. 2017. "About the Endocrine System." Endocrineweb. http://www.endocrineweb.com/ endocrinology/about-endocrine-system

"Science of Psoriasis: Genes and Psoriatic Disease | National Psoriasis Foundation." 2017. *Psoriasis.Org*. https://www. psoriasis.org/research/genes-and-psoriatic-disease

Sears, Dr. 2017. "Standard American Diet (SAD) | Ask Dr. Sears." *Ask Dr. Sears | The Trusted Resource for Parents*. http://www.askdrsears.com/topics/feeding-eating/ family-nutrition/standard-american-diet-sad

Shostak, Sara. *Exposed Science: Genes, the Environment, and the Politics of Population Health*. Berkeley, CA: University of California Press, 2013.

"Speak Your Inner Truth with the Fifth Chakra." 2017. *The Chopra Center*. http://www.chopra.com/articles/ speak-your-inner-truth-with-the-fifth-chakra

Smith, Gina. *The Genomics Age: How DNA Technology Is Transforming the Way We Live and Who We Are*. New York: AMACOM, 2005.

Snyder, Laurence H., and Paul R. David. *The Principles of Heredity*. 5th ed. Boston: D. C. Heath, 1957.

"Spinal Stenosis – Mayo Clinic." 2017. *Mayo Clinic*. http://www.mayoclinic.org/diseases-conditions/ spinal-stenosis/basics/definition/CON-20036105

Stucke, John. "Exposure to Toxins Can Alter DNA WSU Epigenetics Expert Finds Evidence Changes Affect Future Generations." *The Spokesman-Review* (Spokane, WA), June 5, 2012.

"The Dr. Weil Blog – Best In Health, Fitness, Recipes, & Natural Remedies." 2017. *Drweil.Com*. http://www. drweilblog.com/home/2012/9/24/6-reasons-to-drink-water.html

"The Future of Well-Being with Deepak Chopra, MD; Deepak Chopra, MD, explores the concepts of universal consciousness and total well-being." Module 39 of the Health Coach Training Program at the Institute for Integrative Nutrition, Minute 17.

"The Hidden Hazards of Microwave Cooking." 2017. Mercola.Com. http://articles.mercola.com/sites/articles/ archive/2010/05/18/microwave-hazards.aspx

"The Major Rule for Eating Fruit." 2017. Mindbodygreen. http://www.mindbodygreen.com/0-4970/The-Major-Rule-for-Eating-Fruit.html]

"This Happened When I Started Drinking Turmeric Golden Milk Before Bed – David Avocado Wolfe." 2017. David Avocado Wolfe. https://www.davidwolfe.com/turmeric-golden-milk-before-bed

"Thyroid Ultrasound." 2017. *Med-Ed.Virginia.Edu*. https://www.med-ed.virginia.edu/courses/rad/Thyroid_Ultrasound/01intro/intro-01-02.html

"Tired Teen? It Could Be a Warning of Bowel Disease." *Daily Mail* (London), April 2, 2013.

Toft, Daniel J. MD, PhD. 2017. "Graves' Disease Overview." *Endocrineweb*. https://www.endocrineweb.com/conditions/graves-disease/graves-disease-overview

"Toxins in Your Fat Cells Are Making You Sick and Bloated! Here's How You Can Cleanse Them! – David Avocado Wolfe." 2017. *David Avocado Wolfe*. https://www.david-wolfe.com/toxins-fat-cells-cleanse

Trainers, Incline, X9i Trainer, X22i Trainer, and X11i Trainer. 2017. "Incline Trainers Treadmills | Nordictrack. Com." Nordictrack.Com. https://www.nordictrack.com/incline-trainers

"Turn on Your Healthy, Happy Genes." *The Buffalo News* (Buffalo, NY), February 21, 2015.

"ULTRA Running Races & Resources | Ultramarathonrunning.Com." 2017. Ultramarathonrunning.Com. http://www.ultramarathon-running.com/

"VFX BODY." 2017. Vfxbody.Com. http://www.vfxbody.com/learn-more/

Vogel, Sarah A. *Is It Safe?: BPA and the Struggle to Define the Safety of Chemicals.* Berkeley: University of California Press, 2013.

Wellness, Health, Balanced Living, and Exercise Fitness. 2017. "Yoga: More Than a Workout – Dr. Weil." *Drweil.Com.* https://www.drweil.com/health-wellness/balanced-living/exercise-fitness/yoga-more-than-a-workout/

Wellness, Health, Balanced Living, Healthy Living, and Q A. 2017. "Are Plastic Containers Unhealthy? – Drweil.Com." Drweil.Com. https://www.drweil.com/health-wellness/balanced-living/healthy-living/are-plastic-containers-unhealthy

Wellness, Health, Balanced Living, Healthy Living, and Q A. 2017. "Do You Green Dry Clean? – Drweil.Com." Drweil.Com. https://www.drweil.com/health-wellness/balanced-living/healthy-living/do-you-green-dry-clean/

Wellness, Health, Health Centers, Aging Gracefully, and Q A. 2017. "Treating Polymyalgia Rheumatica? – Drweil.Com." *Drweil.Com.* http://www.drweil.com/health-wellness/health-centers/aging-gracefully/treating-polymyalgia-rheumatica/

Wellness, Health, Mind & Spirit Body. 2017. "Anemia – Dr. Weil's Condition Care Guide." *Drweil.Com.* http://www. drweil.com/health-wellness/body-mind-spirit/heart/ anemia

Wellness, Health, Mind & Spirit Body. 2017. "Elevated C-Reactive Protein – CRP – Symptoms, Causes & Treatments." *Drweil.Com.* http://www.drweil. com/health-wellness/body-mind-spirit/heart/ elevated-c-reactive-protein-crp

Wellness, Health, and Mind & Spirit Body. 2017. "Ulcerative Colitis – Dr. Weil's Condition Care Guide." Drweil. Com. https://www.drweil.com/health-wellness/ body-mind-spirit/gastrointestinal/ulcerative-colitis/

Wellness, Health, Mind & Spirit Body, and Autoimmune Disorders. 2017. "Epstein-Barr Virus, Epstein-Barr Symptoms | Dr. Weil." *Drweil.Com.* https://www. drweil.com/health-wellness/body-mind-spirit/ autoimmune-disorders/epstein-barr/

Wellness, Health, Mind & Spirit Body, and Autoimmune Disorders. 2017. "Lupus – Dr. Weil's Condition Care Guide." *Drweil.Com.* https://www.drweil.com/health-wellness/body-mind-spirit/autoimmune-disorders/ lupus/

Wellness, Health, Mind & Spirit Body, and Autoimmune Disorders. 2017. "What Is Fibromyalgia? Fibromyalgia Treatment – Dr. Weil." *Drweil.Com.* http://www. drweil.com/health-wellness/body-mind-spirit/ autoimmune-disorders/fibromyalgia/

Wellness, Health, Mind & Spirit Body, and Pregnancy Fertility. 2017. "Preeclampsia – Dr. Weil." *Drweil. Com.* http://www.drweil.com/health-wellness/ body-mind-spirit/pregnancy-fertility/preeclampsia/

Wellness, Health, Mind & Spirit Body, and Q A. 2017. "What Is Leaky Gut? – Ask Dr. Weil." Drweil.Com. http:// www.drweil.com/health-wellness/body-mind-spirit/ gastrointestinal/what-is-leaky-gut/

Wellness, Health, Mind & Spirit Body, and Stress Anxiety. 2017. "Reduce Stress – Dr. Weil." *Drweil.Com.* http:// www.drweil.com/health-wellness/body-mind-spirit/ stress-anxiety/ten-ways-to-reduce-stress

"What Are the Common Side Effects and Interactions of Thyroid Medication?" 2017. *Naturalendocrinesolutions.Com.* http:// www.naturalendocrinesolutions.com/articles/ common-side-effects-interactions-thyroid-medication/

"What Are Nightshade Vegetables? – Dr. Axe." 2017. *Dr. Axe.* https://draxe.com/nightshade-vegetables/

"What Is BPA? Should I Be Worried About It? – Mayo Clinic." 2017. Mayo Clinic. http://www.mayoclinic. org/healthy-lifestyle/nutrition-and-healthy-eating/ expert-answers/bpa/faq-20058331

"Why We Got Fatter During the Fat-Free Food Boom." 2017. *NPR.Org.* http://www.npr.org/ sections/thesalt/2014/03/28/295332576/ why-we-got-fatter-during-the-fat-free-food-boom

"World Birth Defects Day." 2017. *Centers for Disease Control and Prevention*. https://www.cdc.gov/features/birth-defects-day/

"You Can Influence Genetic Inheritance of Disease; Living Naturally with Olwen Anderson." *Tweed Daily News* (Tweed Heads, Australia), October 5, 2013.

Zakhari, Samir. "Alcohol Metabolism and Epigenetics Changes." *Alcohol Research: Current Reviews* 35, no. 1 (2013): 6+.

Zallen, Doris Teichler. *To Test or Not to Test: A Guide to Genetic Screening and Risk*. New Brunswick, NJ: Rutgers University Press, 2008.

Zonderman, Jon, and Ronald Vender. *Understanding Crohn Disease and Ulcerative Colitis*. Jackson, MS: University Press of Mississippi, 2000.

CPSIA information can be obtained
at www.ICGtesting.com
Printed in the USA
BVHW04s1700150718
521674BV00008BB/102/P